Tennis Today

Second Edition

Glenn Bassett
University of California at Los Angeles

William Otta
Saddleback Community College
Mission Viejo, California

Christine Shelton
Smith College
Northampton, Massachusetts

Series Editor
Bob O'Connor, Ed. D.

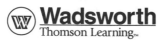
Wadsworth
Thomson Learning

Australia • Canada • Denmark • Japan • Mexico • New Zealand • Philippines
Puerto Rico • Singapore • South Africa • Spain • United Kingdom • United States

Publisher: Peter Marshall
Editorial Assistant: Keynia Johnson
Project Editor: Matt Stevens
Print Buyer: April Reynolds
Permissions Editor: Robert M. Kauser
Production: Fritz/Brett Associates Inc.
Interior and Cover Designer: Harry Voigt Graphic Design

Copyeditor: Susan Defosset
Illustrator: Carole Lawson
Cover Image: Emily Pipas, Smith College
    Tennis Team. Courtesy of photographer
    David Roback and Smith College
Compositor: Pat Rogondino
Printer/Binder: Webcom Ltd.

Printed in Canada

1 2 3 4 5 6 03 02 01 00 99

Library of Congress
Cataloging-in-Publication Data
Bassett, Glenn
  Tennis today / Bassett, Glenn, William Otta,
Christine Shelton. -- 2nd ed.
    p. cm. -- (Wadsworth's physical education series)
    Includes index.
    ISBN 0-534-35835-7
    1. Tennis. I. Otta, William. II. Shelton, Christine.
III. Title. IV. Series.
    GV995.B39 2000
    796.342'2--dc21
                                99-16332

Wadsworth/Thomson Learning
10 Davis Drive
Belmont, CA 94002-3098
USA
www.wadsworth.com

International Headquarters
Thomson Learning
290 Harbor Drive, 2nd Floor
Stamford, CT 06902-7477
USA

UK/Europe/Middle East
Thomson Learning
Berkshire House
168-173 High Holborn
London WC1V 7AA
United Kingdom

Asia
Thomson Learning
60 Albert Street #15-01
Albert Complex
Singapore 189969

Canada
Nelson/Thomson Learning
1120 Birchmount Road
Scarborough, Ontario M1K 5G4
Canada

This book is printed on acid-free
recycled paper.

Contents

Wadsworth's Physical Education Series

Aerobics Today, by Carole Casten and Peg Jordan

Aqua Aerobics Today, by Carol Casten

Badminton Today, by Tariq Wadood and Karlyne Tan

Golf Today, 2nd edition, by J. C. Snead and John L. Johnson

Jazz Dance Today, by Lorraine Person Kriegel and Kim Chandler-Vaccaro

Racquetball Today, by Lynn Adams and Erwin Goldbloom

Swimming and Aquatics Today, by Ron Ballatore, William Miller, and Bob O'Connor

Strength Training Today, 2nd edition, by Bob O'Connor, Jerry Simmons, and J. Patrick O'Shea

Tennis Today, 2nd edition, by Glenn Bassett, William Otta, and Christine Shelton

Volleyball Today, 2nd edition, by Marv Dunphy and Rod Wilde

The Series Editor for Wadsworth's Physical Education Series

Dr. Bob O'Connor received his B.S. and M.S. degrees in physical education from UCLA and his doctorate from U.S.C. His 40-year teaching experience includes instruction in physical education courses for tennis, weight training, volleyball, badminton, swimming, and various team sports, as well as classes in teaching methods. Internationally, Dr. O'Connor has been an advisor to several Olympic programs in weight training and swimming. He was among the first to popularize strength training for all athletic events. Dr. O'Connor has written extensively in the fields of physical education and health.

Preface

In this edition of *Tennis Today*, we have updated the earlier edition and have added three new chapters. The new Chapters 15 and 16 incorporate up-to-date information on nutrition and diet. If you are playing tennis for its fitness outcomes, you will certainly want to increase your fitness in the other important health area—nutrition. Chapter 17 is also new, and includes essential material on fluid replacement and heat-related problems for the tennis player.

We have also added new photos of strength training for tennis. Additionally, Chapter 13 has been updated to include a new section on preventing injury. It has been said that half of recreational tennis players have some arm troubles. These can generally be avoided with proper fundamentals and modern rackets, which are designed to reduce the vibrations of the ball contact that often are absorbed in the arm and elbow.

We hope you like the additional information and that it will make your playing experience even more enjoyable.

How to Use This Book

This book is designed to be used by every tennis player—from the beginning to the advanced tournament player. The basic fundamentals are the same for all. As you advance, you can add another technique or bit of finesse to your swing.

We must walk before we can run. So in tennis we must learn to swing properly before we can hit the ball. We must be able to hit the ball over the net before we can think about placing the ball where we want it. Then we must be able to place the ball before we can think about developing a strategy.

Some players advance very quickly and will be able to think about strategy very early in their playing careers. But players at every level must be concerned about the continual perfection of their fundamentals.

As you read this book, you will be able to see the "whole." You can then select the parts you need to practice to perfect your game at your level of play. This is what psychologists have taught us about sport—work from the whole back to the part, from the overview to the fundamentals. This is the approach we have taken in writing this book.

The 1–2–3–4 Method

This teaching method is a simple 1-2-3-4 approach to teaching the backswing, the step, making contact with the ball, and the follow-through for each shot. This 1-2-3-4 count system will make it simple for you to master the fundamentals of each tennis stroke.

The Drills

After you read a chapter on a fundamental of the game or on strategy, drills will be suggested to you. They will be more fully described and illustrated in Chapter 14. Some drills are appropriate only for beginners, but most drills used by the professionals can also be used by advanced beginners because the fundamentals of the game are similar at beginning and advanced levels of play. For example, practicing a "down the line" or a cross-court shot or working on a volley are done with the same drills for every level of tennis. It is just that the higher-level players are able to hit the ball harder, lower, and with more accuracy than the beginning-level player.

Some beginners are so eager to get into playing a game that they want to reduce the time they spend on drills. But college and professional players practice drills for hours each day. This is how they become so proficient. This is why they enjoy the game more when they play.

There is no substitute for practicing tennis through the drills. Just remember that there is just as much fun in hitting a shot correctly and placing it properly in a drill as there is in winning a point in a game.

Acknowledgments

The development of this text could not have progressed without the helpful criticism and suggestions from colleagues. We gratefully acknowledge the reviewers of this edition: Kathy Jones, Arizona State University; Jonathan Nelson, Northern Michigan University; and Jim Powers, Lorain County Community College. We would also like to acknowledge our colleagues who reviewed the first edition: Duane Klueh, Indiana State University; James LaVanche, University of Dayton; Margie Laney-Lazarine, University of Texas, Arlington; Jo Ann Otte, Weber State College; Thomas Pennewell, Central Michigan University; Bob Rump, Grossmont College; Dick Van Voorhis, Cypress College; and Eloise Wiertel, Ball State University.

Grateful thanks to Christine Wells for her input in the nutrition, diet, and mental conditioning chapters. Her extensive work in these areas has been a major contribution to the book.

Glenn Bassett
William Otta
Christine Shelton

1 *Introducing Tennis*

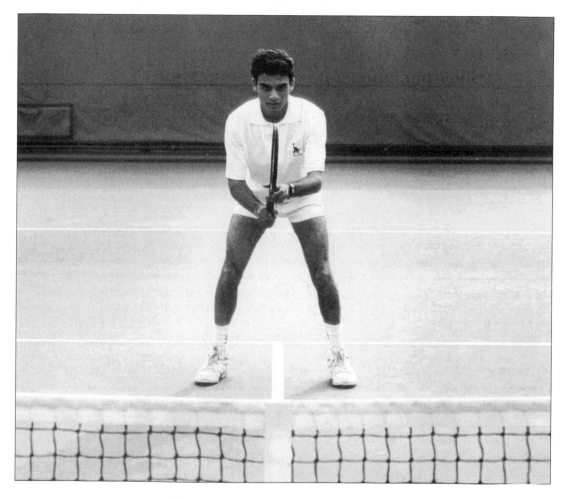

Outline

History of the Game

The ancient Greeks and Romans played a game in which they batted a ball back and forth with their hands. But much closer to our modern game of tennis was a French game of the 1300s in which the nobles used wooden paddles to hit a ball to each other. The game found its way to England but was not popular until the late 1800s, when a portable court was invented. With this invention, the popularity of the game spread around the world. It was first played in the United States in 1875 in Newport, Rhode Island, now the home of the Tennis Hall of Fame.

Over the centuries, it has been variously outlawed as a waste of time, an undignified pastime, an interference with the warlike skill of archery, and, because of the gambling on the matches, an unsavory game. But between these negative periods it was thought of as an ideal amusement or even a game only for noblemen and kings.

The game was first played on grass lawns, which is the reason that, until 1975, the official name of the major tennis organization of the U.S.A. was the United States Lawn Tennis Association. The word "Lawn" has now been dropped from the association's title, since tennis has long been played on clay, concrete, asphalt, and, indoors, on carpet and other surfaces.

Tournaments, both professional and amateur, are held in most countries of the world. The Davis Cup matches teams of men from many countries in an elimination tournament. The Wightman Cup is a similar tournament for women. Major tournaments, such as the Wimbledon in England and the U.S. Open in New York, are well known around the world. And tennis is now again an Olympic sport.

Over the last century, the game of tennis has evolved from a sedate backyard pastime to a highly competitive sport requiring the ultimate in physical and mental abilities—the agility of the basketball player, the mental alertness and intelligence of a football quarterback, and the stamina of a long-distance runner. Today's tennis could be described as a "power" game, one that takes courage, intelligence, and top physical conditioning in order to compete effectively.

The Court

The tennis court is marked for both singles and doubles play. It is 78 feet long. The singles court is 27 feet wide, and the doubles court is 36 feet wide. Lines mark the service areas next to the net. Each service area is 13 ½ feet wide and 21 feet deep.

Grass Courts

The British Open Championship at Wimbledon is the only major tournament played on grass today. A grass court forces players to become more aggressive

**Dimensions and areas
of the court**

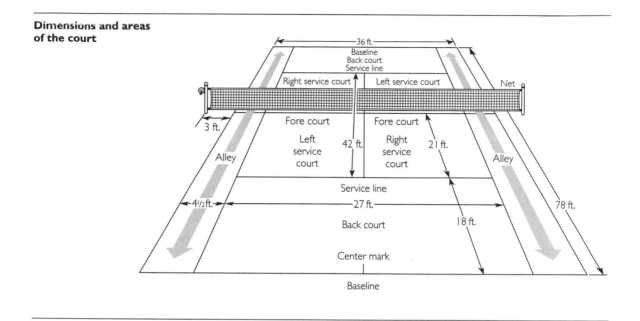

and to come to the net more often so as to reduce the chances of bad bounces from the grass surface. The constant maintenance required of mowing and rechalking the lines is a disadvantage. Moreover, as a tournament is played, the grass becomes thinner and more sparse. And, of course, dampness makes the court unplayable.

Hard Courts

The initial cost of hard courts, made of concrete, asphalt, or similar surfaces, is higher than for any other type of court, but the upkeep is minimal, and balls bounce consistently and faster on this type of surface.

Soft Courts

Generally made of dirt or clay, soft courts are the most common type of court in the world. The game played on soft courts is slower, because the ball bounces higher. Upkeep is a problem, since the surface must be smoothed and packed daily and the lines rechalked or swept daily.

The Game

The tennis *match* begins after one player flips a coin or spins a racket. The player who decides to spin the racket informs the opponent of whatever identi-fying mark is on the racket. For example, a Wilson racket has a "W" on the end of the handle. The opponent can then call "W" or "M" (an upside-down "W").

The racket may be spun on the ground or in the hand. The other player calls one of the sides of the racket, just like heads or tails, and the winner gets his or her choice of whether or not to serve or which side of the court to defend.

The server then takes a position behind the baseline and to the right of the center mark on the baseline. The serve is into the opposite service court. If the opponent does not return the serve, the server wins the point. If the serve is returned, the players rally until one of them has hit into the net, out of bounds, or has missed returning a shot that landed in his or her court.

There are at least four points in a game, at least six games in a set, and three to five sets in a tennis match. There are a minimum of four points in a game, and the winner must win by two points. To win a set, you must win at least six games, and the winner must win by two games or play a tiebreaker. In most tournaments, the winner of the match must win two out of three sets. In major men's tournaments, the players may have to win three out of five sets.

The *game score* is called in large numbers (15, 30, 40) to differentiate it from the *set score*, which is scored in low numbers (1, 2, 3, etc.). A zero score is called *love*. (The term was apparently an English misunderstanding of the French *neuf*, or *neuve*, meaning "beginning," or a mistranslation of another French word, *l'oeuf*, meaning "egg." Indeed, Americans sometimes use the term "goose egg" to mean zero.) The first point is called 15, the second 30, and the third 40. If you win the fourth straight point, it is simply called *game*. The 15, 30, 40 scores might have come from early betting on the points, in which the

Table 1.1

If Server Has Won	If Receiver Has Won	The Score Is
1 point	0	15–love
0 points	1	love–15
1 point	1	15–15 (15 all)
2 points	0	30–love
0 points	2	love–30
2 points	1	30–15
1 point	2	15–30
2 points	2	30 all
3 points	0	40–love
0 points	3	love–40
3 points	1	40–15
1 point	3	15–40
3 points	2	40–30
2 points	3	30–40
3 points	3	deuce
4 points	0, 1, or 2	game to server
0, 1, or 2	4	game to receiver

✓ Checklist for Scoring

1. When a player has not scored a point in a game his or her score is called *love*.
2. The first point in a game is called *15*, which is sometimes abbreviated as *5*.
3. The second point is called *30*.
4. The third point is called *40*.
5. If the score is tied at 40 or any point thereafter, it is called *deuce*.
6. When a player has scored one point after a deuce score, it is his or her *advantage*. This is sometimes shortened to *ad*. A score of *ad in* means that the advantage is in the serving court. *Ad out* means that the advantage is out of the service court—that is, with the receiver.
7. The foregoing scores are called the *game score*.
8. The *set score* is called using the numbers 1 through 6. The server's score is called first.
9. The winner of a set must win six games and be two games ahead of the loser.
10. If the set is tied at six games each, a tiebreaker will be played.

---

first point was worth 15 *sous* (pennies), the second worth 30 *sous*, the third worth 45 *sous*, and the game worth 60 *sous*. The 45 was later shortened to 40.

The server's score is called first. So if the server has two points and the receiver has one, the game would be called *30–15*. If it is tied at 30, it is called *30 all*. If the server wins the next point, the score is *40–30*. If the receiver evens it up, the score is *deuce*, meaning the two players (deuce players) have equal scores. When one of the players scores another point, it is called *advantage*. If the advantage is the server's, it will be called *ad in* (advantage in the serving court). If the receiver has the advantage, it is *ad out* (advantage out of the serving court). The game will continue with ad ins, deuces, and ad outs until one person with the advantage wins another point and it is game.

Some tournaments are using *no ad* scoring. In this type of scoring, the winner must win only four points, so there will be no ads. In no ad scoring, the points are called 1, 2, 3, 4 rather than 15, 30, 40, and game. If the score gets to 3–3, the receiver has the choice of courts in which to receive the serve.

The set score is also called with the server's score first. So a score of 2–4 would indicate that the server has won two games and the opponent has won four. The set won't be completed until the winner has won at least six games and is ahead by at least two games, so the score might be from 6–0 to 6–4. Until recently the players had to play until one had won by two games, so scores such as 10–8 or 15–13 were not uncommon, and occasionally a score of something like 45–43 would show up in a tournament. Today the *tiebreaker* is generally played to eliminate such long sets. It is played when the score is 6 all.

The Tiebreaker

The United States Tennis Association has adopted the twelve-point tiebreaker. The player wins who first gets seven points and is at least two points ahead. The first server is the player who would have served first in the next set. He or she will serve the first point from the right court. The second player will then serve points 2 and 3 from the left, then right courts. Then Player A (the first player) serves points 4 and 5 from the left, then right courts. Player B serves the sixth point from the left court. Then the players change ends. (Rest time is not allowed.)

Player B next serves from the right court. Player A serves the following two points from left and right, and the rotation continues. Play continues until one player is ahead by two points. They will change ends every six points. When the tiebreaker is decided, the player who did not serve first will serve first in the next set.

In doubles play, tie-breaking scoring is similar. The team whose turn it was to serve the next game serves first. Player A1 serves from the right court. Player B1 serves from the left, then the right court. Player A2 serves from left, then right. Player B2 serves from the left. Then they change courts. Play continues as in singles.

The Server

The server is allowed two serves to get the ball into the opponent's service court. The server must stand behind the baseline and must not touch the line or the court beyond it until the ball has left the racket on the serve. Stepping on or across the line is called a *foot fault* and invalidates the attempted serve.

The server serves from the right court—also called the *forehand court* for right-handed players—whenever the score is even, that is, during the first service of the game and when the score is love–30, 15 all, 30 all, or deuce. For this reason, the right side is also sometimes called the d*euce court.* Service is made from the left court—also called the ad or *backhand court*—on love–15, 30–15, 40–30, and advantage points.

The serve is made to the diagonal court. The lines are in bounds, so "liners," or balls that land on the lines, are good. Balls that land outside the lines are "out." If the player serves from the wrong court and points have been scored, there is no penalty. Once the error is discovered, the server begins serving from the proper court for whatever the score is at that time.

The rules state that the player must toss the ball and hit it before it reaches the ground. Technically, the ball can be hit by an underhand, sidearm, or the common overhead serve. The ball can be tossed up and caught with no penalty—as long as the server does not swing at it. (Swinging and missing is a *fault.*) So it doesn't pay to swing at a poorly tossed ball. Just catch it.

If the server steps into the court before the ball has left the racket, or if the serve misses the service court or hits his or her partner (in a doubles match), it is a fault. Two faults (called a *double-fault*) result in a point for the receiver.

**Position of
the server**

S1 = Singles server
to forehand
or deuce court

S2 = Singles server
to backhand or
add court

D1 = Doubles server
to forehand
or deuce court

D2 = Doubles server
to backhand or
add court

**Serving targets for
right-handed receiver**
1,4 = to forehand
2,5 = at receiver
3,6 = to backhand

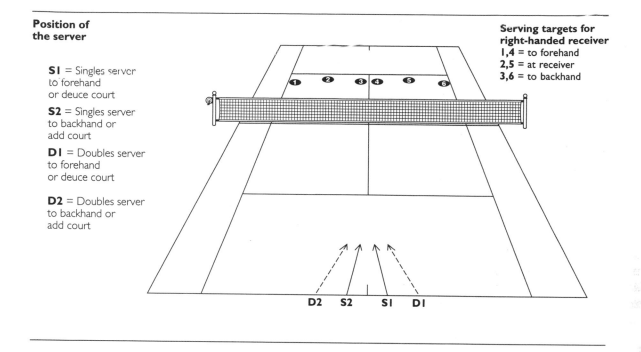

If a served ball hits the net and goes into the proper court, it is called a *let*
ball, and the server is allowed to serve that ball again. If the receiver is not
ready when the ball is served, he or she can also call a let ball. Furthermore, a
let ball can be called if there is some sort of interference with the game such as
a ball coming from another court or a loud noise that disrupts concentration. In
this case the whole serve is replayed so that the server has two chances to get
the serve in.

Receiving the Serve

The serve can be received from any position on the court. The only rule is that
it must hit the ground before it is returned. Although you can take time to get a
stray ball out of your way, it is not good sportsmanship to unduly delay the
server's second serve and thus disrupt the server's rhythm.

Changing Ends of the Court

Players switch ends of the court to equalize whatever disadvantage one player
has, such as sun in the eyes, shade, or wind. Ends are changed after every odd-
numbered game: first, third, fifth, and so on. The same pattern of changing
continues into the second and third sets. So if a set is ended on an even-

numbered game, such as 6–2, players do not change ends until after the first game of the next set.

You Score a Point When:

1. The ball lands in your opponent's court but is not returned into your court. Even if the ball hits a fence or other object after landing in your opponent's court, it is your point. It is also your point if the ball does not go between the net posts on the return shot.
2. The ball bounces twice on your opponent's court.
3. Your opponent catches any hit ball before it bounces—even if it is obviously out of the court. The ball must be given the chance to drop into the playing court.
4. Your opponent hits the ball twice on his or her side of the court or "carries" the ball on the racket rather than making a good, clean hit. (Hitting the ball with the wood or metal part of the racket, however, is legal.)
5. Any part of your opponent, his racket, or clothing touches the net while the ball is in play.
6. Your opponent hits the ball before it crosses the net. (It is permissible to follow through over the net after the ball has been hit.) The one exception that allows a player to reach over the net is when the ball has already bounced on his or her side of the net but then bounces back to your side because of wind or backspin.
7. The ball hits any part of your opponent except the racket.
8. Your opponent throws the racket at the ball (even if the return is successful).
9. Your opponent deliberately interferes with your making a shot. If the interference is unintentional, it is called a let ball and is played over. If the interference is caused by your ball hitting a ball lying on your opponent's side of the net, you score a point, because each player is responsible for removing such balls.

Doubles Play

In doubles play, partners alternate games for service. So if you serve the first game, your partner will serve the third, and your opponents will serve the second and fourth games. For the second set, either partner can begin the serve, even if he or she was the last to serve in the first set.

In receiving a serve, the partners decide before a set which one will receive all the serves in the deuce court (the forehand court). The other will receive all serves in the ad court (the left, or backhand, court).

Etiquette in Tennis

Tennis has long been known as a game for ladies and gentlemen. Good manners are expected. The standard for etiquette in tennis is higher than that of some other sports, such as hockey.

Before the Match

When you are walking to or from your court, be sure that you don't bother other players. If you have to cross a court to get to your court, wait until a point is finished, then cross the court next to the fence at the rear of the back court area.

Be certain that you have all of your equipment, including a second racket, at courtside. You are not allowed to leave the court after a match begins—not even if you break your racket. You should also have a beverage container in case you get thirsty.

Before the match, introduce yourself to your opponent if you are not acquainted. Spin the racket to determine who will serve and which sides will be defended, then start your warm-up.

Complete all of your warm-up before beginning the set. Both players should have taken all their practice serves. You are not allowed more practice serves once the match has begun.

Etiquette in Serving

In serving, always have at least two balls ready. Call the score before each first serve. After every point, all balls should be returned to the server—not just rolled to his or her side of the net. If a ball has gone onto another court, ask the players for the ball. A simple "Thank you" or "Ball, please" lets them know that there is a ball on their court.

If a serve is obviously a fault, just call it out and let it go by. Don't hit it after calling it out. If your opponent returns a serve that you thought was out, you must play it.

Etiquette During Play

When there is no umpire, tennis players generally give their opponent the benefit of any doubt on a call. If you are not sure about a ball being on the line or out, you give the point to your opponent.

Tennis players are expected to make all the calls on their side of the court if there is no umpire. If you double-hit or carry the ball, or if you touched the net, you should call it on yourself. If a ball is out, say "Out" immediately. You don't need to call balls in; just play them. When in doubt about a ball, assume it is in, and play it. Always give your opponent the benefit of the doubt.

Always accept your opponent's calls without arguing or grumbling.

If a ball rolls on your court and disturbs your play, call a let, and play the point again.

If there is a ball on your side of the net, and the ball you are rallying hits it, you lose the point because you should have removed the ball before play began.

If you are playing on a court next to other courts in use, refrain from critical comments. This includes criticizing your partner in doubles. Don't do it.

Etiquette as a Spectator

Spectators should not talk, applaud, or do anything that might distract a player while a point is in play. Intense concentration is required of tennis players. Applaud good points only after the point is completed.

In tennis, the game is to be won fairly.

Summary

1. The game of tennis is a popular international game with a long history.
2. The court is marked for singles or doubles play.
3. The scoring is such that:
   - At least four points must be scored to win a game.
   - At least six games must be won to win a set.
   - In tournaments, two or three sets must be won to win the match.
4. A tiebreaking game is played when the set score is 6 all. In a tiebreaker, the winner must win at least seven points and be ahead by two.
5. The server is allowed two attempts (plus any let serves) to get the ball into play by serving into the proper court.
6. A player wins a point when:
   - The opponent does not hit the ball back before it has bounced twice.
   - The opponent catches a flying ball before it hits the ground.
   - The opponent hits the ball out of bounds.
   - The opponent touches the net while the ball is in play.
   - The ball hits any part of the opponent except the racket.
   - The opponent throws the racket.
7. Etiquette and good manners have long been expected on the tennis court.

2 *The Equipment*

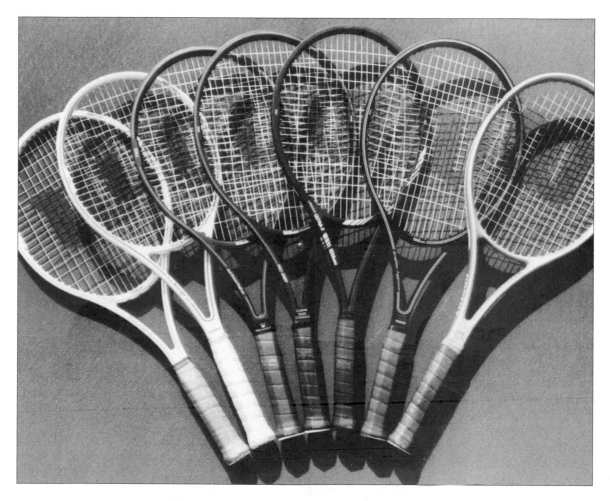

Outline

Buy a good racket. Yes, you can save money by purchasing an inexpensive one to try it out, or, if you are a beginner, to see if you even like the game. The trouble is that bad rackets can contribute to a bad game and to arm injuries, resulting in discouragement not only with the racket, but with tennis. Also, bad rackets wear out quickly, and your initial economy is wasted after all. People who play a great deal of tennis generally own two rackets of similar weight, and they alternate them so the action stays similar as the rackets wear. Also, should one break, they have the other to play with until the first is repaired.

Rackets

Rackets may be stiff, *whippy* (flexible), light, heavy, or light or heavy in the head. There are different weights and different grip sizes. Racket heads may be round, oval, or oversized. Characteristics of these various features are as follows:

- Stiff rackets generally control the ball better but transmit less power.
- Flexible (whippy) rackets generally give more power and a better serve.
- Rackets with oversized heads and a larger "sweet spot" are usually better for beginners.
- Heavy rackets usually aid in hitting the best ground strokes.
- Light rackets move faster for volleys and serves.
- Head-heavy rackets hit the ball harder.

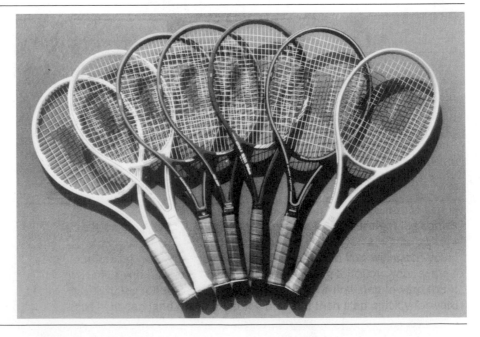

A sampling of the wide variety of racket styles

**The widths of
rackets vary**

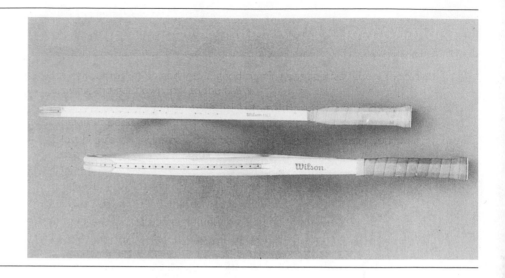

- Head-light rackets can be moved faster for serves and volleys.
- Wooden rackets give the most feel and absorb shock. But today few wooden rackets are sold.
- Metal rackets move faster and last a long time but transmit shock. Magnesium is the most common metal used in rackets today.
- Graphite rackets are for people who hit hard and swing through the ball. Their major advantage is that they are very light.
- Composite rackets (various combinations of graphite and fiberglass) are common today. The fiberglass takes some of the shock out of hitting the ball. The better rackets are 70 to 80 percent graphite. The less expensive are about 30 percent graphite and are acceptable only for the beginner and the weekend player.
- Ceramic rackets are strong and stiff.
- Titanium rackets are light but have little vibration, so they are less likely to cause *tennis elbow*, a condition in which there are injuries to the muscles or connective tissues in the back of the arm just below the elbow. The racket's *sweet spot* (the area in which the ball is best controlled) is also quite large.

It's better to begin with a light racket, something that weighs between 13 and 13 ¼ ounces. Medium-weight rackets run between 13 ¼ to 13 ¾ ounces, and heavy rackets are 14 to 15 ounces or more. The heavier the racket, the stronger you should be to play it, because over a series of sets the extra weight will begin to strain your arm and hand. When the extra-weighted racket is used in the backhand swing, it can contribute to tennis elbow.

To check a racket for balance, hold it horizontally and lightly at the throat—the widened area between the handle and the head—to see which way it wants to tip. Remember, head-heavy rackets hit harder, but head-light rackets are easier to whip around and handle.

The heads of rackets vary

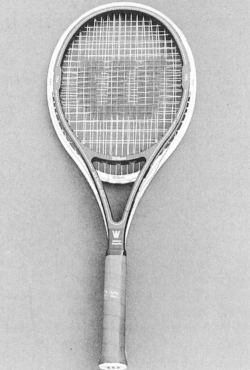

The Handle

As if you don't have enough decisions to make, there are different shapes and sizes of handles from which to choose. Sizes run from 4 to 5 inches in circumference. Some people measure from the lifeline of the palm of the hand to the top of the ring finger to decide the correct size. Another way is to grip the racket and make sure a half-inch of handle shows between your fingers and the base of your hand. Other people make their decision strictly according to comfort and feel.

A handle grip that is too small will allow the racket to turn easily in your hand when you are playing, which will throw off your shots. Then, in trying to correct for the small grip, you may hold the racket too tightly and thus lose the relaxation that is so important.

Strings

String, material, and tension strength should be selected based on your game. Most advanced players like *gut* material because it can be strung more tightly and seems to provide a better feel of the ball. It also holds the ball on the racket longer and more securely. It is more expensive initially, however, and it

> ✓ **Checklist for Buying a Racket**
>
> 1. Beginners should buy less expensive rackets that have been strung at a factory rather than at a pro shop.
> 2. The oversized head is generally better for beginning-level players.
> 3. Stronger people can buy a stiffer racket. Weaker people should use a more flexible (*whippy*) racket.
> 4. Select a racket that has a handle grip comfortable for you.
> 5. Select a racket with a grip large enough to allow about a half-inch of space between your fingers and the base of your hand. Most beginners buy rackets that are too small, allowing the racket to slip in their hands.
> 6. Seek the help of a tennis expert rather than an ordinary salesperson. The fit of the racket is very important, since it determines whether the handle will slip in your hand and whether or not you can control the racket

tends to loosen and sag when there is a great deal of moisture in the air. Few players actually require cat gut strings in order to play their best game. The synthetic strings, such as nylon, are ideal for beginners and most intermediates. They're strong, durable, and inexpensive, and they react to the ball almost as well as gut. Their major disadvantage is a tendency to break without warning. Gut shows wear, so you can anticipate upcoming trouble.

Both nylon and gut string can be strung to different poundages. The more tightly strung your racket is, the more rebound the ball will get from strings. Most top players using gut have their rackets strung tightly (60 to 65 pounds) in order to get maximum power on each shot; but remember, these are players who can control the ball. A new player with synthetic strings will probably find 45 to 55 pounds more satisfactory.

String also varies in its gauge. Thicker-gauge strings last longer but do not give the feel of the thinner strings to a racket.

Beware of blaming all your playing deficiencies on the racket. Tennis clubs are full of intermediate players who spend hundreds of dollars every year buying "new, improved" rackets in an attempt to get a "new, improved" game.

Balls

The type of tennis balls you use can make a difference in your game. Obviously, old balls lose some of their fuzz and some of their bounce. Both are vital factors in the way the ball plays off your racket and off the ground.

The balls with the truest bounce, the type used in tournament play, get most of their bounce from the compressed air inside them. Beginners get more play out of "pressureless" balls that get their bounce out of the rubber rather than the compressed air.

Tennis balls come in two types: championship and heavy-duty. The championship type is faster and ideal for slow courts. Heavy-duty balls are ideal for fast courts and for playing at higher altitudes.

Save your old balls. You can practice with old balls as long as they have some bounce left. Keep a sack of them nearby while practicing to save yourself some of the monotonous task of retrieving balls.

Rejuvenating-type cans that repressurize the balls can be bought to keep your old balls bouncier. Fuzzing machines can restore the balls' nap. Also, you can keep the older balls in pretty good shape by running them through a clothes washer and dryer occasionally.

Footwear

Shoes

Shoes for playing tennis should be light but have thick soles and a deep tread to help you stop quickly. Reinforced toes are important because of those sudden stops that occur in the game; they keep the front of the shoe from wearing out prematurely. Make sure the shoe is constructed well, gives you good support, and has a strong arch that won't break down with constant pounding. The constant pounding can contribute to "overuse" injuries in the feet, ankles, and knees. For this reason, a good shock-absorbing sole is important.

Players who have narrow feet seem to like the models that lace to the toes, because the shoe can be made tighter on the ball of the foot. If you have an average foot, the shoes that lace only partway down may be fine. When you lace your shoes, always start from the bottom and tighten the laces at each eyelet. This gives you a much better fit than just pulling the laces tight from the top.

Canvas shoes are good for hot-weather playing. The canvas "breathes," so it keeps your feet drier, which not only contributes to comfort but also helps you avoid infections such as athlete's foot. Leather and synthetic materials last longer, but shouldn't be used in hot weather because they keep the heat and moisture trapped inside the shoe. For cooler weather, all materials are good.

Socks

For comfort and to avoid blisters, try wearing two pairs of socks instead of one. Ideally, the inside pair should be cotton and the outer pair wool. This is the best combination for foot comfort and sweat absorption. If you like the new, partially synthetic socks, wear them on the outside; but remember, man-made materials generally don't absorb perspiration.

✓ *Checklist for Comfortable Footwear*

1. If you are subject to blisters, wear two pairs of socks.
2. Lace your shoes from the bottom up each time you put them on. Putting on your shoes and pulling at the top of the laces is not enough. Proper fit requires that you tighten each lace from the bottom to the top, then tie the shoes.
3. Select shoes specially designated for tennis. Each type of athletic footware is designed for a specific activity. Jogging shoes are not appropriate for tennis.
4. Select shoes with proper arch supports. Cheap shoes usually do not have such supports.
5. If you have foot problems, have an orthopedist or other medical person design orthotic devices to wear in your shoes.
6. Additional cushioning can be gained by using special rubberized insoles in your shoes.

Clothing

Tennis outfits are highly attractive, and new designs, colors, and imaginative trim are regularly introduced on the market. Since white reflects heat, though, you should choose it (or another light color) over dark colors, however dramatic their look, as the dark colors absorb heat and can drain your energy on a warm, sunny day. Also, cotton will keep you cooler. As with shoes, man-made fabrics tend to hold in the heat and do not let perspiration evaporate.

Some of the attractive new clothing is not specifically designed for the game. In their attempts to ride the tennis trend, a few manufacturers have merely redone a standard line of clothing and called it tennis wear. These lines cannot accommodate the stretching and reaching that tennis demands. Conversely, some lines have special elastic or expandable inserts, slits, pleats, and other devices that give your body total freedom of movement. Before you buy, make sure the clothing won't bind, cramp, or chafe you.

In addition to dresses or shorts and tops for women and shorts and shirts for men, tennis wardrobes should also include a good warm-up suit. These outfits are ideal for playing in cooler weather as well as for warming up. They also help to prevent chills after a hot, sweaty game. For cool weather, you should also have a couple of sweaters, wearing both of them while you warm up and then removing them one at a time as you work up a sweat.

Other Equipment

You'll notice that many players have a special bag in which they carry not only rackets and balls but additional gear for their game. These bags generally contain sweat bands for the wrist and sometimes for the forehead, a hat or visor, a towel, a handkerchief to tie around the neck, especially on hot days, a change of socks, shoes, or clothing, Bandaids, tape, soap, deodorants, Gauzetex or powder to apply on slippery grips, extra balls, chewing gum, candy, sweaters or jackets, ball pressure cans, and even a jug filled with water or another type of thirst-quenching liquid.

Summary

1. Proper equipment is essential in order to play well, avoid injuries, and enjoy the game more.
2. Rackets come in varying sizes and in several types of material. A good professional or teacher can help you to determine which type of racket and string is best for you.
3. Your shoes and socks are very important. Proper fit reduces the chances of blisters. Proper tread gives you better traction.
4. Your clothes can be colorful and attractive, but they should be practical and allow you to move effectively and let your body dissipate heat.
5. Be sure to have water or another thirst-quenching type of beverage available when you play or practice.

3   *The Grips and the Footwork*

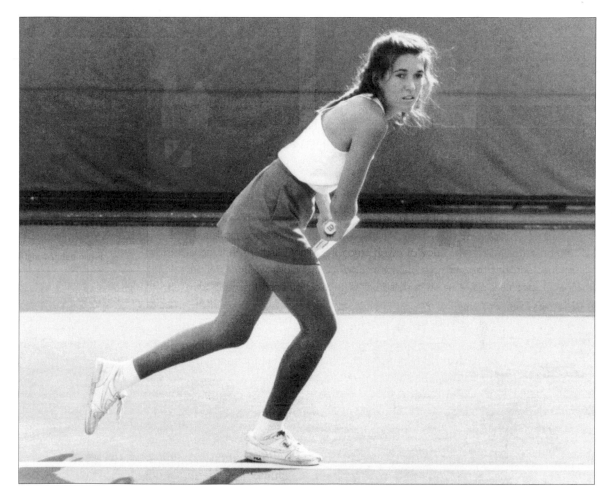

Outline

The fundamentals are the key to success in every sport at every level. When you see a tennis player talking to his or her coach during a tennis match on television, you may think they are plotting some exotic strategy when, in fact, chances are the coach is telling the student to bend the knees more, to watch the ball, or to complete the follow-through. Whether you are a beginner or a pro, you must always pay strict attention to the fundamentals.

Eliminating Variables

For consistency in any sport, you must eliminate variables. For example, as a beginner, try to keep your forehand grip exactly the same on every forehand shot and your backhand grip exactly the same on every backhand shot. Your footwork should be consistent. The more things that you can do the same on each shot, the greater will be your consistency.

Another way to eliminate variables is to bend your knees for low shots. If you bend at the waist for low shots you bring different muscles into play. So for every shot, whether it is waist-high or just above the ground, use the same arm swing and vary only the flexion of your knees to bring you to the level of the ball.

As you move from a beginning to advanced level of play, you will gain more control of your body and therefore can add variables to make special shots. For example, you might wish to change your grip to get more topspin on a forehand shot.

The Grip

A proper grip is fundamental because it connects your body to your racket. If your body does everything perfectly in a swing but the racket is held wrong, your ball will not go where it is aimed.

Your grip should change depending on where you plan to contact the ball. If you were to hit every ball, forehand and backhand, when it was in front of your belly button, you would never need to change grips. But since most players contact the ball before it gets to their forward foot, they either have to change the grip slightly for the forehand and backhand, or they have to change the angle of their wrists. Changing the angle of the wrist should be avoided, since it adds another variable to the swing.

If you have received any instruction in tennis, you've no doubt been told how to hold your racket at least 100 times. So let's discuss it for the 101st time so we can start out together. Some of you may be familiar with the information that follows, but most of you will find a surprise or two.

If you want to play well and win, one of the most important requirements is to be able to feel the ball on your racket. No feel, no control. It's that simple. To that end, the racket is held with the fingers and not the hand! First, spread your fingers comfortably, take the racket in the handshake position with the racket held primarily by your index and middle fingers, both relaxed. If you hold these fingers too tightly around the handle, you will lose the feel of the ball, and the continual tension and strain will soon tire your hand, arm, and shoulder. Also, relaxed fingers help you move the racket faster when you have to shift to a backhand shot.

Forehand

There are three types of forehand grips: the eastern, the western, and the continental, which is really a forehand-backhand compromise. Each grip has its advantages and disadvantages.

The forehand grip begins with what is commonly called the shake-hands grip. (Technically, it is called the eastern forehand grip.) With the racket head perpendicular to the ground, your wrist should be in the same position as it would be in shaking hands. The top bone in your index finger will be directly behind the handle. The racket is held with your index and middle fingers on the back of the racket and your thumb on the front. The end of the handle is braced under the fat part of your hand behind your little finger. It is not held in the palm of your hand, so in this respect it differs from shaking hands, which is done with the palm of the hand. The tennis racket is held more with your fingers.

The racket should be gripped rather loosely until just before contact with the ball. Holding it too tightly can tire you because of the tension in your arm and shoulder. And with a tight grip, you won't be able to feel the ball on your racket as you stroke it toward your target.

Eastern forehand

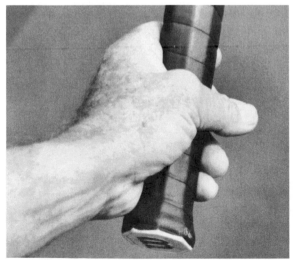

Left-handed

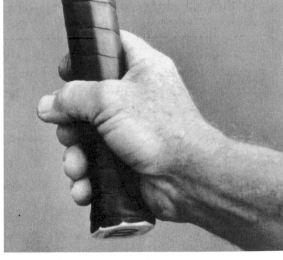

Right-handed

Continental forehand

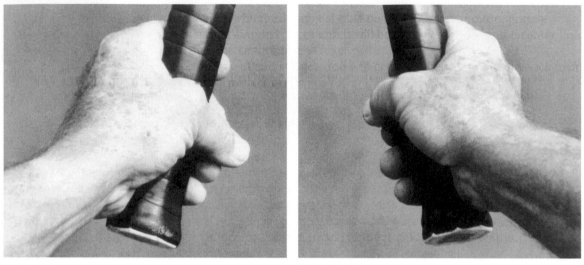

Left-handed   Right-handed

The eastern forehand grip is best for beginners and intermediate players. It provides feel, control, and the right angle to the racket head when swung properly. Most of the American pros use this grip.

A more advanced grip, sometimes used by some top players, is the continental grip. In this grip, the palm of the hand is moved more to the top of the racket, allowing the player to use the same grip for the forehand and backhand shots. It would be a perfect grip if all shots were hit in the center of the body, but power and accuracy dictate that the ball should be hit in front of the body whenever possible. The continental is the favorite grip of many Australian players. It is also the preferred grip of players who like to slice their backhand shots.

A third grip, the western forehand grip, is often used by advanced players playing on clay courts. In this grip, the palm is moved under the racket, allowing the player to give the ball more topspin. The western forehand is not recommended for beginners or intermediates. Players who like to rally from the back court sometimes use this grip. Some of the European pros prefer it as their basic grip.

Backhand

The most commonly used backhand grip is the eastern backhand. In this grip, the hand is moved more to the top of the handle, while the thumb braces the back of racket, allowing the player to impart more power to the ball.

If you use the eastern forehand and backhand grips, you will be able to hit the ball in front of your body while keeping the angle of your wrist the same. So by changing your grip, you can eliminate a body variable. Of course, those who use the continental grip won't have to change grips, but if they choose to

Western forehand

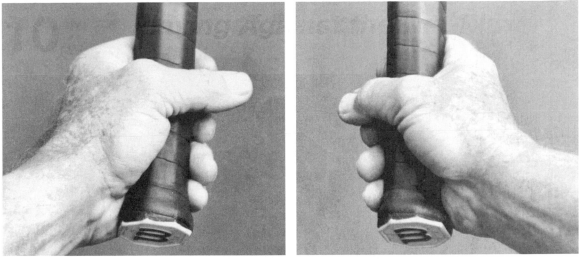

Left-handed   Right-handed

hit the ball in front of them, they will have to change their wrist angles slightly—adding a variable.

The top players actually do change their grips slightly for different kinds of shots, but beginners should avoid this by sticking to the eastern forehand and backhand grips for all shots.

A powerful backhand shot is the two-handed backhand, which is discussed in Chapter 5.

Eastern backhand

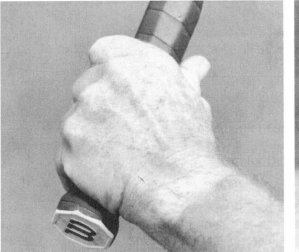
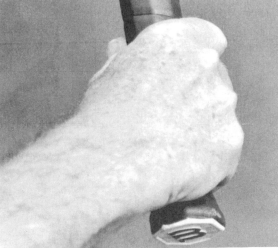

Left-handed   Right-handed

Two-handed backhand

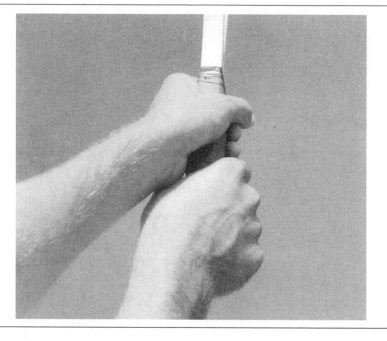

✓ *Checklist for Grip Before and During the Swing*

1. Hold the racket in both hands so that you can change to whichever grip you will need—forehand or backhand.
2. Be ready to choke up on the grip if it helps you to control the ball.
3. Spread your fingers comfortably on the racket handle.
4. Hold the racket handle in a relaxed manner until you feel the ball.
5. Firm your grip upon contacting the ball—but don't squeeze too tightly.

Ready Position

The ready position in tennis is much like the ready position in other sports. The infielders in baseball and the defensive backs in football use similar ready positions. To receive most shots, you should be a step behind the baseline, with your weight on the balls of your feet and your knees bent. Your torso should be forward. Both hands should be on the racket, and your eyes on the ball.

Footwork

Your footwork should get you to the ball in a proper hitting position. Some people prefer to run to the ball, then set up for the swing. This method can work whether the ball is near or far. If the ball is close, most players like to shuffle or skip sideways to the ball.

The sprint

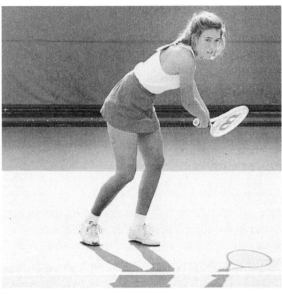

Beginning sprint

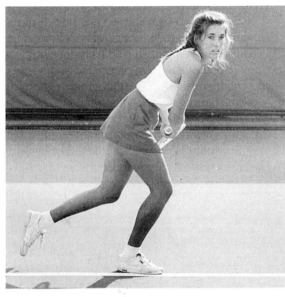

Sprint

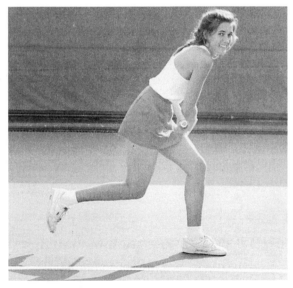

Sprint completed

Sliding footwork

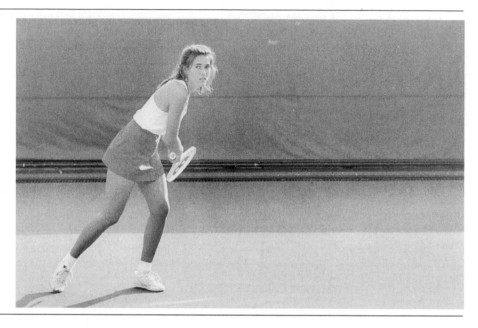

Start your footwork with your eyes. Watch the ball as it comes off the strings of your opponent's racket, and start in the direction that it is going. For the backhand, get your racket back as you slide sideways. Face the net and keep your eyes on the ball as you slide.

Crossover footwork

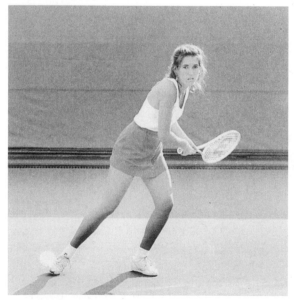

Slide toward backhand side

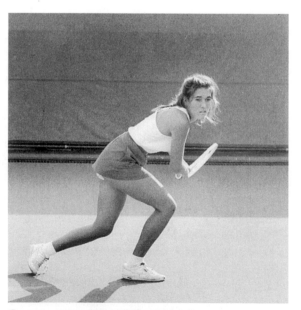

Crossover step as backswing is completed

When you are ready to hit, take your full backswing and step into the ball with your forward foot (the right foot for right-handed players). As you complete your swing, bring your rear foot forward and slide back to the center of the court.

The principles are the same for the forehand. Backswing with the weight on your racket-side foot (right foot for right-handers), then put your weight on your forward foot (left foot for right-handers), and swing through the hit. Then bring your back leg forward and return to the center of the court.

An alternative step is to cross over (your right foot past your left, if going left). This step also allows a full weight shift to the forward foot.

✓ Checklist for Footwork

1. Keep your feet moving—never stand still.
2. Use your eyes. Try to see the ball as soon as it comes off your opponent's racket.
3. Glide to the ball while you continually watch it.
4. Cross over with your front foot just before contact.
5. After hitting the ball, recover quickly, and balance the court by taking a position that will cut off your opponent's angle shots.

Four-Count System for Tennis Strokes

Years of teaching have shown the authors that a simple four-count procedure can help students develop the proper timing for tennis strokes:

1. The short backswing
2. The step forward
3. Making contact with the ball
4. The follow-through

Following this procedure for each shot will simplify the learning for tennis players at all levels.

Summary

1. Fundamentals are for everybody. Not only should the beginner be totally concerned with fundamentals, but every top player must concentrate on the fundamentals of the sport.
2. Because tennis strokes require very fine coordination, it is important to eliminate as many variables in the swing as possible. A slight change in the grip or an excessive bend at the waist can throw your whole shot off its mark.

3. The eastern forehand is the most common forehand grip. In this grip, the top bone in your index finger is directly behind the racket.

4. The eastern backhand is the most common backhand grip. In this grip, your thumb rests behind the racket.

5. The eastern forehand and backhand grips will allow you to hit the ball before it crosses the plane of your body, helping you to gain power and control in your ground strokes.

6. Always attempt to get into the ready position before your opponent hits a shot.

7. Proper footwork is essential to approach the ball properly.

Drills for the Beginner

1. *Feeling the Ball on the Racket.* Hold the racket with your palm facing upward so that the flat part of the racket head is parallel to the ground. Place a ball on the sweet spot—the middle of the strings. Just bounce the ball upward from the racket. How many times can you hit it upward without letting it hit the ground? Get used to feeling the ball bounce on your racket.

2. *Bouncing the Ball on the Court.* Turn your palm so that it faces the ground. The racket head should be parallel to the ground. Now bounce the ball from the ground to your racket. How many times can you bounce it without missing? When you become proficient at bouncing the ball in one place, walk along and bounce the ball off the ground.

O f the forehand grips discussed in Chapter 3, the eastern forehand grip is recommended. To achieve this grip, just "shake hands" with the racket, making sure that the top bone in your index finger is behind the racket. The base of the handle of the racket should rest under the fat part of your hand, behind the little finger. And the racket should be held primarily with the index and middle fingers behind the racket and the thumb in front.

Four-Count System for Forehand Stroke

As mentioned earlier, the four-count system explained in this book is both simple and effective. It works for every stroke: forehand, backhand, approach shot, volley, and serve. In this chapter, we apply it to the forehand. Though the instructions may seem complicated, they are not. Once you begin to follow them, your body and natural reflexes will carry you through automatically.

You can easily pick out the times and places that are throwing off your natural forehand stroke. The single most important thing to remember is the 1-2-3-4 rhythm of the forehand and what happens with each count.

Count One: The Backswing

If you wait to start your backswing until the ball gets to you, or even until it crosses the net, you are also going to wait a long time to develop a winning game. Even the best players with the fastest reflexes start their backswings as soon as they see the ball coming off their opponent's racket. The backswing should be finished and in place by the time you get into position to return the

The ready position for all ground strokes

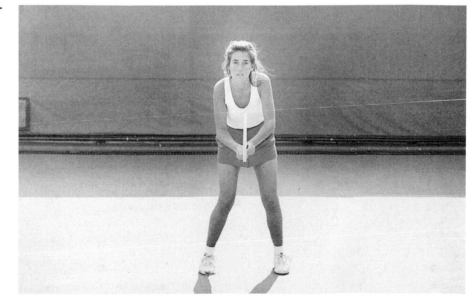

4   *The Forehand*

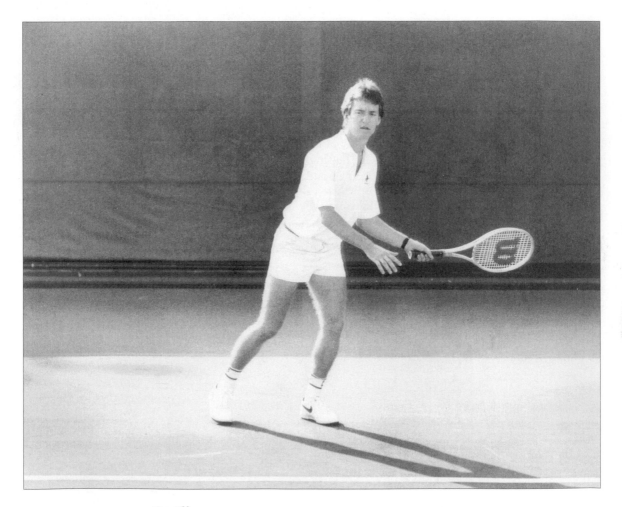

Outline

Count One:
The backswing

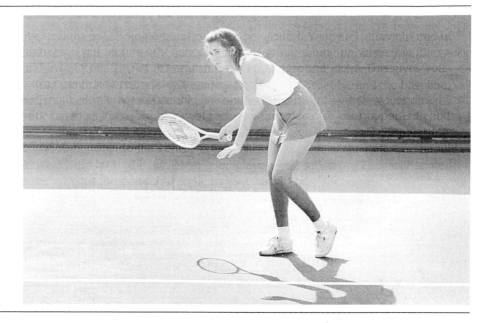

ball. For beginners, intermediates, and even those advanced players who are having trouble meeting the ball in front of them, *take a short, straight backswing*.

You can run faster and more easily to the ball when your racket isn't making useless arcs in the air, or isn't so far back that you're out of control and off balance as you move across the court. After you have mastered the straight-back backswing and are more advanced, you can use a circular backswing if you like.

The straight-back backswing starts with the racket head moving backwards perpendicular to the ground—with the racket head and not the arm moving first. To do this, bend your wrist back a little from your arm, so the head of the racket actually leads the backswing. This will give power to your return. During this part of the backswing, your arm is also slightly bent at the elbow and fairly close to the body.

Take the racket head back a little lower than your wrist for normal or low-bouncing balls, but slightly higher than your wrist for high-bouncing balls. If the ball is going to have a great deal of bounce, lift your entire arm slightly.

For intermediate and advanced players who use the circular backswing, the racket head should go back higher than your elbow. The advantages of the circular backswing are more rhythm and more power, but you have less control, and they take more time.

Many players make the mistake of moving their elbows too much. At the start of the backswing, the elbow is in front of the hip. At the end of the backswing, it should have moved to only the back of the hip and a few inches away from it. At the end of the backswing, the arm should still be relaxed and bent slightly at the elbow and wrist. The right, or *hitting*, shoulder should be turned slightly back. (Left-handers should transpose these instructions.)

The left hand, for right-handed players, has an important job in the back-swing. Too many players let it flop around instead of using it as an important part of the backswing. Ideally, the left hand stays on the racket, in a cradling position, for 6 to 12 inches at the start of the backswing. This helps guide the racket back and also forces the left shoulder around just enough to afford the maximum power and control. Too much body turn for beginners and interme-diates can deplete that control and power by forcing you into a cramped posi-tion. Advanced players, of course, begin to turn sideways more and more as timing improves.

When your left hand slides away from the racket, it should move out natu-rally and easily toward the oncoming ball. This helps balance your body and gives you the hand-eye communication with the ball that helps you keep it in front of you.

Your body should be in a slightly curved (that is, a comma) position during the backswing. Your knees should be slightly bent for waist-high shots. They should be flexed a great deal for low shots. Your body should be slightly bent forward from the waist. And your head should be bent forward so your eyes are as much on a level with the ball as possible. Try not to bend over with your back, but rather use your knees to get down. This helps you see the ball and get under it. Think of making a triangle, with your head, left hand, and right hand forming the angles of the triangle. This is important!

☛ **TIP:** Try not to strangle the racket handle in a hammerlock. Hold it tightly enough for control but loosely enough to get the feel of the ball.

Count Two: The Step

Just before you want to make contact with the ball, *step forward with your for-ward foot*, making sure that you don't overstride or throw yourself off balance. Your head and body will move forward naturally, and the weight of your body will shift from your back leg to your front one. Push off your back leg to get onto your front leg. Make your body lean a little out over your front leg. When possible, make sure your front foot steps in the direction you want your ball to go.

This step forward gives you more of an "opened-up" position. The racket now moves farther back so that it is 180 degrees, or perpendicular, to the net. Letting the racket head get farther around than that can give you more power but can affect your control. Advanced players can master it, but beginners and intermediates should work more on maintaining control.

Although your elbow is still slightly bent and relaxed, the step forward will automatically straighten your arm a little and move your elbow farther away from your right hip. Your wrist is still laid back a little from your arm, and the racket head is lower than the spot where you plan to hit the ball, and either perpendicular to or slightly turned toward the ground, or *closed*. If you are plan-ning a topspin return, the racket head should be closed.

The other arm remains in front of you, still pointing at the ball and still relaxed. Meanwhile, keep your head forward—don't lift it.

Count Two:
The step

☛ **TIP:** Shift your weight from your back leg to your front leg, making sure your body doesn't shift too far forward and throw you into an off-balance reaching position.

Count Three: Making Contact with the Ball

There are two major places for your racket head to meet the ball. If you want to return the ball cross-court to your opponent, your racket should connect with the ball before it reaches an imaginary line extended from your front foot. Hit the ball when it is 6 to 12 inches on the net side of your front foot. If you want the ball to go straight, or down the line, hit it 6 or less inches in front of that front foot. *Always make contact before the ball has passed that imaginary line that is an extension of your front foot.*

When rallying or practicing, try to hit a high percentage of forehand cross-courts, because this helps you learn how to hit the ball in front of you.

When the racket head starts forward to meet the ball, it moves out and away from your body, carrying your elbow out and away. (This is called an *inside-out* hit because your racket starts close and moves out from your hip.) Your arm is slightly bent at the start of the forward movement, but it straightens as it approaches the ball. By the time you hit the ball, the arm holding the racket is nearly, but not totally, straight. The racket head should be moving upward on a diagonal, so it will lift the ball up and over the net. On high-bouncing balls, use less lift, but make sure you use some. (Many players beat themselves by frequently putting the ball into the net and losing points.)

Count Three: Making contact with the ball

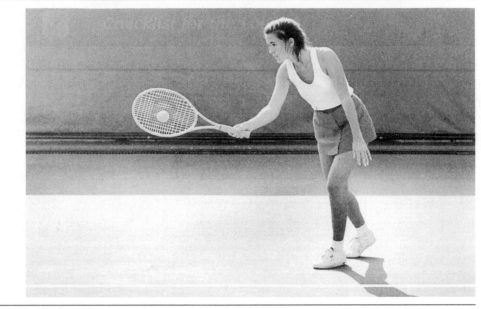

Intermediate and advanced players can think about contacting the ball in one of three angles: closed, open, or perpendicular. If you want to return the ball with a lot of topspin or hit a high-bouncing return, hit it with the racket face closed (turned slightly toward the ground). On normal-bouncing balls that you want to return flat and with power, keep the racket head vertical (perpendicular to the ground).

At the moment of contact, the racket head should be even with your wrist and arm. Wrist, arm, and racket should be parallel to the net if you want your shot to go down the line. If you want to place your shot cross-court, your racket head should have gone past the point where it is parallel to the net.

Your fingers tighten naturally on your grip at the moment of contact. They should grip the racket securely enough so it doesn't twist or turn in your hand but not so tightly that you lose the feel of the ball. Make sure your head is down and your eyes stay as level with the ball as they can. Your head will automatically move forward, but should not move up.

Your shoulder and hips also move forward with the stroke, but your rear leg should stay back, the heel lifting from the ground and the toe dragging. Try to keep that rear foot touching the ground. If it lifts completely, it can throw you off balance and affect your return.

For *low balls*, just bend at the knees. For *high balls*, take your backswing high and swing straight through at the ball. The other option is to let the ball drop to waist level, then hit it.

**Count Four:
The follow-through**

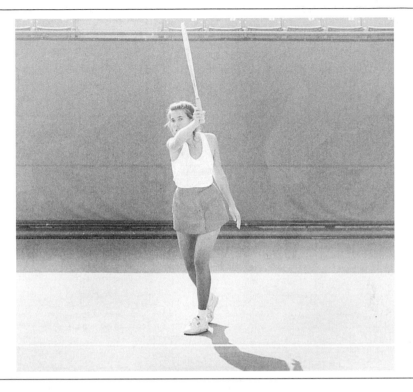

Count Four: The Follow-Through

Follow-through on your forehand stroke gives you accurate placement and power. It is the payoff, the most important part of the entire swing. To accomplish it, you must keep your racket on the ball in a straight line for 6 inches to a foot after you meet it. This gives the ball direction and power and helps you to "feel" the shot.

The arm holding the racket moves the racket head through the ball in an absolutely straight movement at this time. Your right shoulder comes forward until it is ahead of your left shoulder. At the finish, your head should still be down. Your right shoulder swings through until it touches your chin and remains there through the finish. The racket finishes higher than your head.

Your legs begin straightening after you have stayed with the ball for 6 inches to a foot. They should be completely straight at the finish, with all of your weight on the front foot. This gives you additional power and a natural topspin. Your head also moves up with your body but continues looking at the ball. If you lift your head too soon, the movement of the racket will be affected, and you will lose that perfect contact with the ball. More advanced players can roll the racket over the ball to give the ball topspin.

The only time you tighten your fingers on the racket grip is during the hit and follow-through. You tighten them only enough to keep the racket from slip-

**The full sequence for
the forehand—right-handed player**

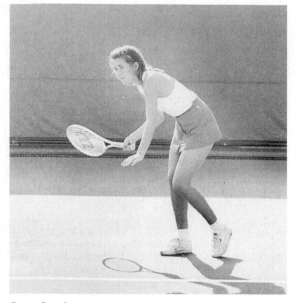

Count One: Running position

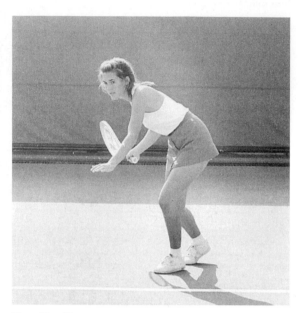

Count Two: The step

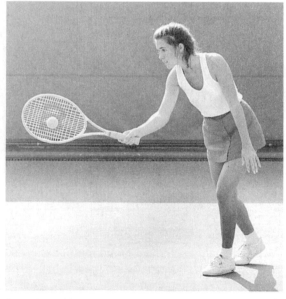

Count Three: Making contact with the ball

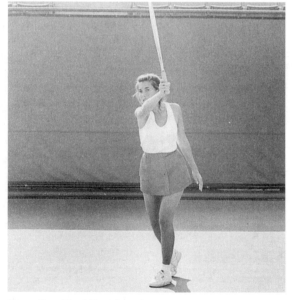

Count Four: The follow-through

**The full sequence for
the forehand—left-handed player**

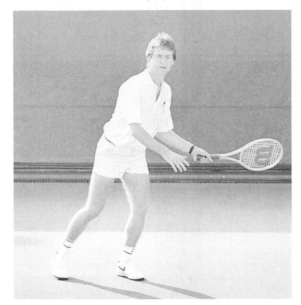

Count One: Running position

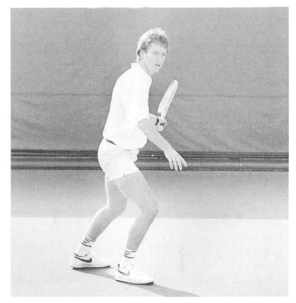

Count Two: The step

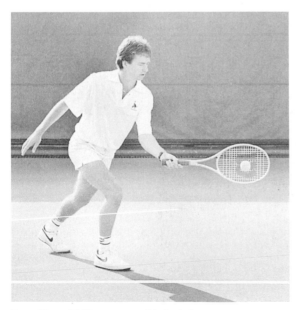

Count Three: Making contact with the ball

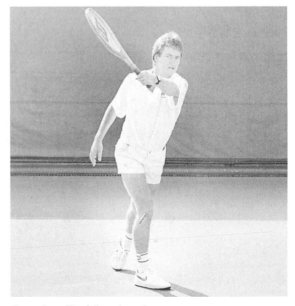

Count Four: The follow-through

> ✓   *Checklist for Forehand—Right-Handed Player*
>
> 1. Keep your racket back and move to the ball.
> 2. Step onto your left leg before contact. Transfer your weight to that leg.
> 3. Make contact with the ball out in front of your left leg.
> 4. Have a strong follow-through. Your right shoulder should touch your chin.
> 5. Hold onto your follow-through for a split second, and then recover fast.

> ✓   *Checklist for Forehand—Left-Handed Player*
>
> 1. Keep your racket back and move to the ball.
> 2. Step onto your right leg before contact. Transfer your weight to that leg.
> 3. Make contact with the ball out in front of your right leg.
> 4. Have a strong follow-through. Your left shoulder should touch your chin.
> 5. Hold onto your follow-through for a split second, and then recover fast.

ping out of your hand or twisting. Remember to keep your fingers relaxed enough to get the feel of the ball all the time it is on the racket.

After you complete the forehand follow-through, you should freeze for a second or two to check yourself and make sure you are balanced. Do this every time you practice, and it will soon become a natural habit you will use in play.

Summary

1. The forehand is the most powerful of the ground strokes. It should be a natural hitting action, yet it must be practiced. As a beginner, just work on the straight backswing. As you progress, you will want to use the circular backswing and put topspin on the ball.
2. Start your backswing as soon as you see the ball leaving your opponent's racket.
3. Step forward and hit the ball before it becomes even with your body.
4. Complete a full follow-through while still watching the ball.

Drills for the Beginner

1. *Hitting Against "Air."* Practice the four-count action described in the chapter for each stroke and serve. Practice your stroke without hitting a ball. You can practice this in front of a mirror at home. Get the feel of leaning into the ball as you hit it, and complete the full follow-through.

2. *The Drop-Serve into a Fence.* With the racket in one hand and the ball in the other, drop the ball, then hit it into the fence after it has bounced off the ground.

3. *Hitting the Slow-Pitched Ball.* Using either a partner or a ball machine, have the ball pitched slowly to the hitting player. Let the ball bounce, then hit it.

4. *Hitting Against the Wall.* There are several drills in which a wall can be used.

   a. Standing about 25 feet from the wall, drop-serve the ball and hit it to the wall, then catch it.

   b. Move farther away from the wall. Now drop-serve, and rally with yourself, keeping the ball in play as long as possible. Try to keep the ball between 4 and 7 feet from the ground. (Since the net is 3 to 3 ½ feet high, you must clear the net, but you should not hit the ball too high.)

   c. As you get better, move farther from the wall, perhaps as far as 40 feet. You will have to get set more quickly, because the ball will return faster than it will when rallying with a partner. If you are 40 feet from the wall, the ball will travel 80 feet between each of your shots. On a court, the ball will travel about 160 feet (the length of the 78-foot court twice).

Drills for the Advanced Beginner to the Expert

On all drills for ground strokes, hit the ball deep. Try to get the ball within 5 feet of the baseline. These drills are discussed further and illustrated in Chapter 14.

1. *Forehand Down-the-Line Ground Shots* can be practiced with the help of a partner or a ball machine. The partner tosses or hits the ball to your forehand, and you hit the down-the-line shot. You can place a target 3 feet inside the sideline and 4 feet inside the back line.

2. *Cross-Court Ground Shots* are practiced the same way—forehand and backhand. For the best practice and better physical conditioning, return to the center of your court after each shot.

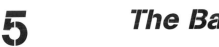

5 The Backhand

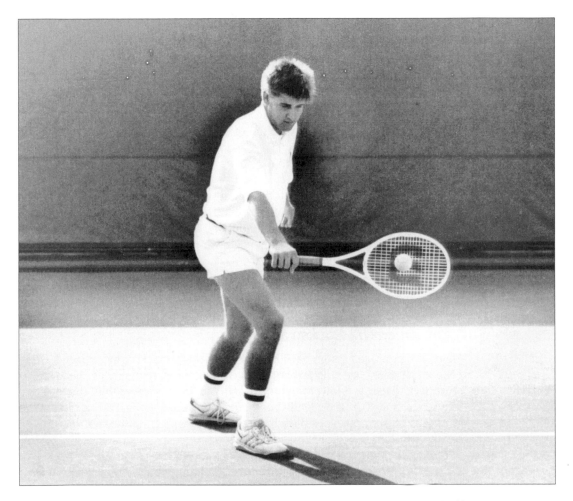

Outline

Tennis, like all racket sports, is a game played from two sides of the body. Without a good backhand, the player is immediately handicapped for 50 percent of the time and will soon be handicapped all of the time as the opponent learns that weakness. Regardless of how strong your forehand is, you cannot hope to "run around" all your backhand shots to return them with your forehand. First of all, it takes too much time to move around to the forehand side to hit them with your forehand, and second, an opponent who is accurate can drive you right off the court with a series of shots you should be handling with your backhand.

There is only one solution: learn the backhand and continue to practice it—against backboards, against friends, against opponents—until it is as good as your forehand. Many players find that after they have learned the backhand properly, it actually becomes their best and strongest stroke.

Of the backhand grips discussed in Chapter 3, the eastern backhand is recommended. Bring your hand to the top of the racket and brace the backside of the racket with your thumb. Now move your weight over the foot that will be forward when making your backhand shot and see if the racket head is perpendicular to the ground.

For the beginner, the backhand movement provides a natural away-from-the-body swing for control and power when meeting the ball. For intermediate and advanced players, the backhand should be as easy, natural, and effective as the forehand because most opponents hit to it often. Consequently, most serious players practice it a great deal.

Four-Count System for Backhand Stroke

Count One: The Backswing

The racket arm does not go back first for the straight-back swing. Instead, the racket head does. The wrist is bent open a little, allowing the racket head to move back ahead and lower than the wrist. The wrist is lower than the elbow. Both elbow and wrist are slightly bent. (For the circular or figure-eight backswing, the racket head goes back higher than the wrist, and the wrist goes back higher than the elbow.)

The left hand (for right-handers) has two important jobs during the backswing. If you are going to change from the forehand grip to the eastern backhand, your left hand cradles and supports the racket approximately halfway up the shaft while you turn the racket approximately one-eighth of a turn. Your thumb can also be placed in a diagonal position on the grip at this time.

The second job of the left hand is to lead the racket back until it is about even with your left hip. The fingers of your left hand are cupped and under the racket at some point between the middle and the top of the shaft. Your left hand stays in that position until you get to the third count of the swing and are hitting the ball.

Turn your body a little sideways to the net with your weight on your left or back leg and knees bent and relaxed. Your eyes should be on a level with the oncoming ball.

Count One:
The backswing

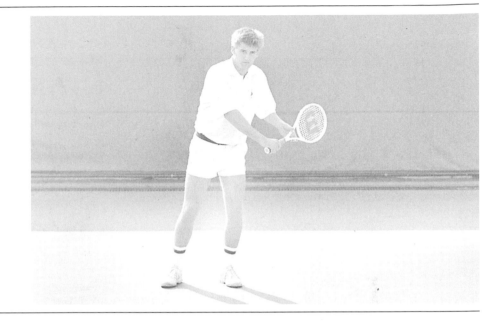

Count Two: The Step

Like the forehand, the correct point of the contact with the ball should be 6 to 12 inches in front of your front foot if you want to hit the ball cross-court, and 6 inches or less in front of that foot if you want to hit it straight down the line.

Judging the speed of the oncoming ball, begin your forward step so that you will contact the ball at the proper distance from your front foot.

Your front foot (which will be the right foot for right-handers) steps in the direction you want the ball to go; all of your body weight shifts from the back foot onto the front one. Be careful not to overstride, throwing yourself too far forward and off balance. Also be sure to shift that weight forward to your front leg to gain maximum stroke power. As you step forward, the racket (with both hands still on it) will automatically go back a bit more, completing your backswing and putting you into a tight, coiled-up position. Some players do get the racket back more than 180 degrees to the net to gain more power, and there is some loss of control for all but the advanced players.

Your racket arm automatically straightens out more as you step forward. Your elbow is still slightly bent and a few inches from your stomach. Your wrist is still bent slightly, and at this point, it allows the racket head to drop slightly so it will connect under the ball during the hit.

Your body moves forward naturally as you step forward, stopping when it is balanced over the forward (right) leg, your head out in front of that leg. Your head does not lift as you swing forward. Your eyes should see only the ball. Although your head does move ahead of the front leg, make sure it does not pull your body too far forward. This could pull you into an off-balance condition that will have you reaching for the ball.

Count Two:
The step

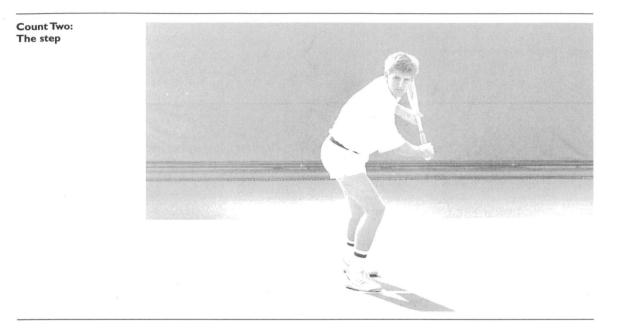

☛ **TIP:** Both hands remain on the racket all the way through Count Two.

☛ **TIP:** Be sure that you are away from the ball. Being too close, which is a common beginner's error, will result in an unwanted slice because you have "crowded" the shot.

Count Three: Making Contact with the Ball

Where you hit the ball and how you hit it is crucial to the backhand. Many players who seem to have the form down perfectly still can't get the ball back accurately or with power. They are hitting too early, too late, or with the racket head in the wrong position and location. Yet the backhand hit should be a natural, easy-flowing movement that gives mastery to the return.

The proper point of contact between the racket head and the ball should be between 6 to 12 inches in front of your front foot if you want the ball to go cross-court, and 6 inches or less if you want the ball to go straight down the line. Remember, if the ball gets past your front foot before you hit, you're late, and you've lost control and power.

Time your contact. Just as your racket arm starts forward, your left hand should finally leave the racket shaft. Your right arm is slightly bent at first but straightens out as the racket gets closer to the ball. By the time you contact the ball, your arm should be almost straight, with the racket parallel to the net.

As you move the racket forward, it moves naturally out and away from your body. The racket is moving upward and forward in a diagonal motion so that it

**Count Three:
Making contact with
the ball**

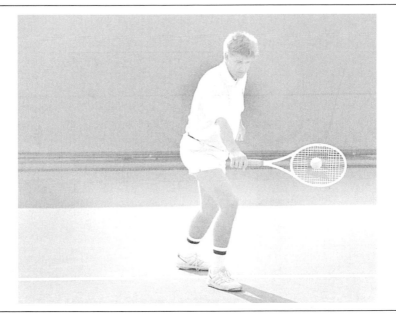

will lift the ball up and over the net. For high-bouncing balls you don't need as much upward motion and can keep the racket closer to parallel with the ground.

For low balls, bend your knees and get down so the racket can get under them. Get the head of the racket below your wrist, and turn your wrist slightly so the top edge of the racket leads. For high balls, adjust the racket so it comes forward above your waist, with the top edge of the racket head leading slightly or at least even with the bottom one.

For cross-court shots, the racket head must connect with the ball when it is slightly ahead of your wrist. Down-the-line shots are made when wrist and racket are in a straight line and parallel to the net.

Tighten your fingers at the moment of contact so the racket won't twist or turn in your hand, but make sure you don't get a hammerlock on the grip and thus lose the feel of the ball.

Your body uncoils naturally as the racket arm swings through the hit, but it does not straighten up until you are in the follow-through phase of the swing. Too many players, even competition-trained ones, develop the bad habit of lifting their entire bodies during this part of the stroke. That jerks the racket up instead of through the ball, and the ball generally ends up in the net or is an easy "put away" for your opponent. Remember to *keep your eyes on the ball* continually from the time it comes into your racket strings until it leaves them. Although your head moves forward, your eyes should stay on the ball.

As you uncoil while hitting, your right shoulder moves forward in the intended direction of your hit, and your hips begin to turn to face the net. Your weight

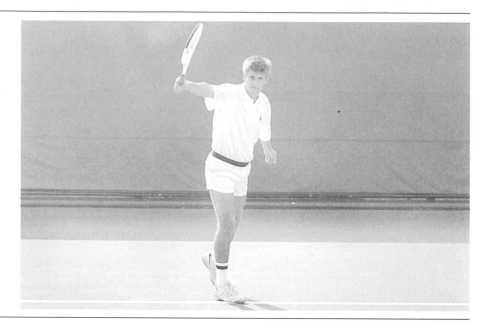

is on the ball of your front foot, and the left toe begins to drag a little, the heel lifting naturally from the ground.

Count Four: The Follow-Through

If you follow through correctly, you greatly increase your chances of making an effective shot. The most important part of the follow-through is keeping the racket head in contact with the ball. If you hold the ball on the racket for 6 inches after contact, you will increase your power, control, and feel.

If you merely brush your racket across the ball, it will probably not go where you want it. So it is necessary to develop the ability to feel the ball with your fingers. When the racket head meets the ball, feel it there, and hold the racket steady and smoothly straight through that 6-inch part of the follow-through. Aim exactly where you want the ball to go.

At the end of that 6-inch movement, your arm and fingers begin moving the racket diagonally up and out. Your intent is to finish with the racket aimed exactly where you want the ball to go, but the natural momentum of the swing will carry it beyond that point. The racket moves across your body and finishes higher than your head.

Your arm rolls the racket slightly over the ball while your arm is straightening. The top edge of the racket head will turn slightly ahead of the bottom edge. Make sure you don't flick or break your wrist and, as a result, lose control of the follow-through stroke.

**The full sequence for
the backhand—right-handed player**

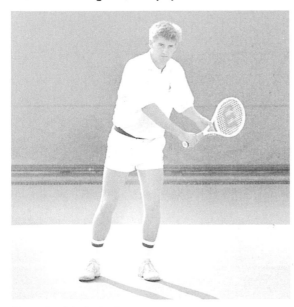

Count One: The backswing

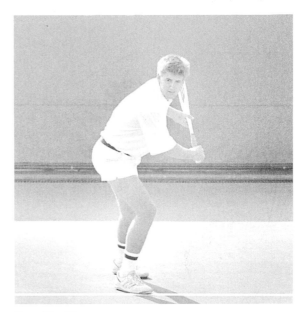

Count Two: The step

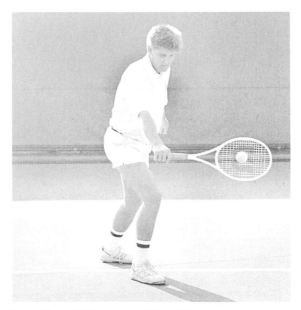

Count Three: Making contact with the ball

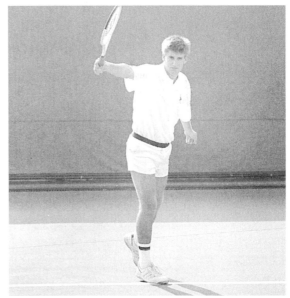

Count Four: The follow-through

**The full sequence for
the backhand—left-handed player**

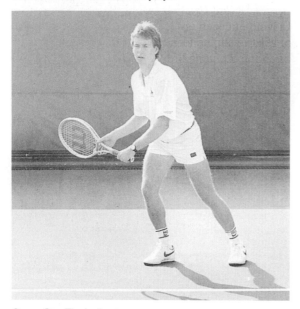

Count One: The backswing

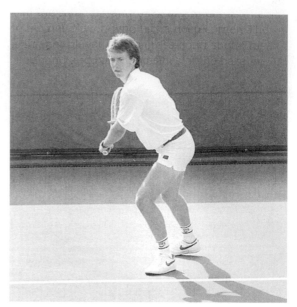

Count Two: The step

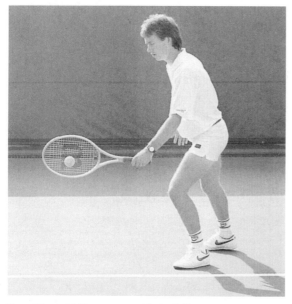

Count Three: Making contact with the ball

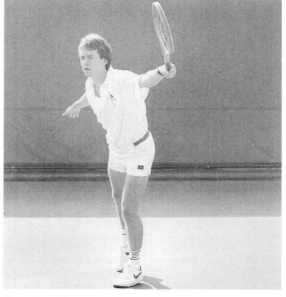

Count Four: The follow-through

✓ *Checklist for Backhand—Right-Handed Player*

1. Get your racket back fast, and move to the ball.
2. Step into the ball, before contact, with your right leg. Transfer your weight to that leg.
3. Hit the ball out in front of your right leg.
4. Use a strong follow-through.
5. Keep your balance, and your follow-through position, for a split second, and then recover fast.

✓ *Checklist for Backhand—Left-Handed Player*

1. Get your racket back fast, and move to the ball.
2. Step into the ball, before contact, with your left leg. Transfer your weight to that leg.
3. Hit the ball out in front of your left leg.
4. Use a strong follow-through.
5. Keep your balance, and your follow-through position, for a split second and then recover fast.

As your hitting arm goes forward, your right shoulder moves forward also until the arm is straight. At that point it moves up and around, opening up your body so you are now facing the net at a 45-degree angle. The arm and shoulder movement together give you the power you need for a strong backhand return. Meanwhile, your left shoulder swings forward a little but always stays in back of the right one. At the finish of the stroke, your right shoulder is higher than your left. Your racket is now higher than your head.

At the very end of your follow-through, all your weight is over your front leg, the back leg dragging a little to maintain your balance. As with the forehand, hold your final position a second or two to check it and make sure you are balanced. Make a habit of checking your final follow-through position. It will become an automatic reflex and a constant reminder to you of the proper form for the backstroke.

☛ **TIP:** Concentrate on keeping the ball on the strings for 6 inches after making contact. This is the single most important part of the follow-through stroke and gives you the drive and feel you need for an effective return.

Backhand Slice

So far we have been working with the backhand *drive*—the shot that gives you both power and depth. Depth is probably the most important advantage you can give your ground strokes. But the *slice* is the most versatile and consistent backhand shot.

The backhand slice should definitely be part of your collection of ground strokes. You will need it a great deal in competition play. For example, when you have to hit a ball on the rise, a slice will put more of your racket strings on that ball and give you more control than a standard drive stroke. That's because the strings are actually coming down on the ball in the slice instead of moving up and across it as in a drive. It's also easier to hit high-bouncing balls with the slice, because you can get your racket head higher and still produce a powerful return.

In addition, the slice can become your backup stroke for those times when your drive isn't working and you've lost confidence in it. When you do lose your backhand drive stroke (and one of those unsolved mysteries to tennis coaches is why it tends to come and go with even the best of players) and are losing points and games and your tennis self-esteem, drop the drive and switch to the slice immediately. Then, as you begin to pick up your confidence—maybe in the same set or match—go back to your drive again. Don't, however, get in the habit of depending upon the slice as your bread-and-butter backhand. It cannot give you the power and depth of the backhand drive.

Even if your backhand drive is working well, there are two times you might want to play the percentages by using your slice. The first occurs when you have an opponent who doesn't like the way the slice return stays low and skips across the court surface. Second is when you are playing someone whose timing becomes confused and can't seem to handle the slice return. In these cases, stay with the slice as long as you can. When your opponent begins to start handling it, then go back to your backhand drive or begin mixing them to keep that opponent confused and off balance.

Another time to bring your slice into play is when your opponent is a so-called hit-and-miss player. The best way to beat such a player is by keeping the ball in the court and "in play." Eventually, this type of opponent will miss a return. A deft combination of drives and slices will confuse the opponent and gain you important points.

Four-Count System for Backhand Slice

Although you must continue the basic 1-2-3-4 count system, there are some bodily variations between the slice and the drive.

Count One: The Backswing

Take the racket head up higher than your wrist before you begin to move it back. The racket head should be more open than it was for the drive. It should tilt back farther and face the sky but still remain above your wrist.

The backhand slice

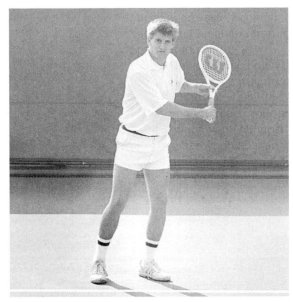

Count One: The backswing

Count Two: The step

Count Two: The Step

When the racket head starts forward, it should either be at the same height or above the ball, not below it and moving up as with the drive. Be sure to step before the hit.

Count Three: Making Contact with the Ball

You can think of your stroke as "throwing" the racket head down at the ball. The racket head actually moves in a downward flight at the oncoming ball. At the moment of contact, the face of the racket closes a little, depending upon how much slice you want. The more slice you need or want, the more open your racket should be. Practice the angles of the racket face until you can master the amount of slice you desire for each situation.

Count Four: The Follow-Through

On the follow-through, the bottom edge of your racket head is still out ahead of the top edge and leads it all the way through to the finish of the slice follow-through. At the finish of the slice follow-through, the racket is generally about head-high. If you can put a great deal of slice on the ball, it can end up higher.

The backhand slice—continued

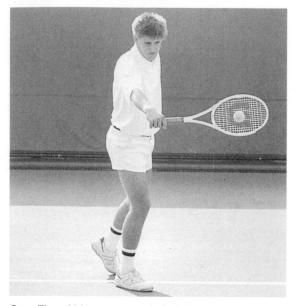

Count Three: Making contact with the ball

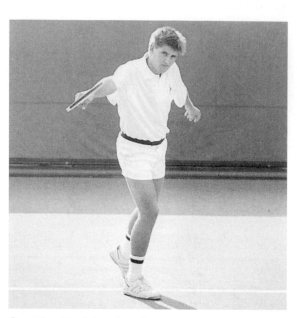

Count Four: The follow-through

Unlike the drive, your hitting arm and your right shoulder do not open up or roll over. You should be able to see the back of your hand on the slice follow-through, whereas you see the palm on the drive follow-through.

Make sure you get the feel of the ball and that you stay with it for that critical 6 inches of control. Also make sure your arm is completely straight after staying with the ball and all the way through to the completion of the follow-through.

Your head stays down throughout the backhand slice. It stays parallel to the ground, forward and out in front of your body.

Finally, on the backhand slice follow-through, when you are hitting high balls, hop a little bit forward and land on your front leg. This helps your balance, prepares you for the return, and gives you additional power and control.

Two-Handed Backhand

If you are small, lack arm strength, or have elbow problems, you may want to use the two-handed backhand. It will give you more power than the one-handed stroke, but you won't be able to reach as far to get a ball on your backhand side. Some people will also have problems when they have to volley with one hand when a shot comes to their backhand side.

The two-handed backhand

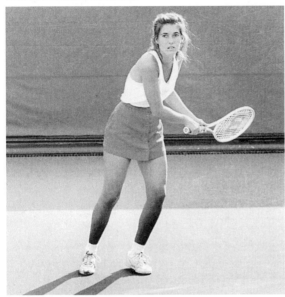

Count One: The backswing

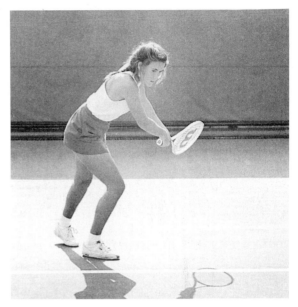

Count Two: The step

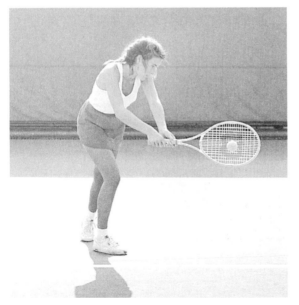

Count Three: Making contact with the ball

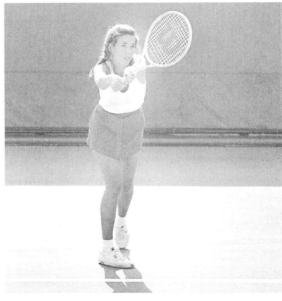

Count Four: The follow-through

The grip for the two-handed backhand is the continental grip—with your right hand lower on the racket and your left hand above it for right-handers. Your footwork is very important. You must get to the point where you can step directly into the ball.

Other Backhand Shots

Some of the better players work on an extreme *backhand topspin*. This is the riskiest of all the backhands, but if the opponent gives you the opening, it could result in a win for you.

The *floater* is a high, hanging slice. It is a slow shot most often used on clay courts.

The *drop shot* is really just a soft floater that barely clears the net.

Summary

1. The backhand must be mastered, because most players will play to your backhand, since it is generally less powerful than the forehand.
2. Get your racket back as soon as possible as you move to the ball.
3. Transfer your weight onto your forward foot as you lean toward the net.
4. Hit the ball before it is even with your body.
5. Use a strong follow-through.

Drills for Players at All Levels

Use the same drills as those in Chapter 4 on the forehand, then add the following drills in which you will combine the forehand and the backhand. These drills are discussed further and illustrated in Chapter 14.

1. *Backhand Down-the-Line Drill.* One player hits a down-the-line forehand, and the other player returns it down the line with a backhand. This is a drill for high-intermediate to advanced players. The drill should be done on one side of the court, then the other, so that each player has a chance to practice both the forehand and the backhand down-the-line shots.
2. *Combination Cross-Court and Down-the-Line Drill.* One player hits only cross-court shots and the other hits only down the line. This drill forces both players to run and hit. It helps your conditioning as well as your stroke development.

6 *The Serves*

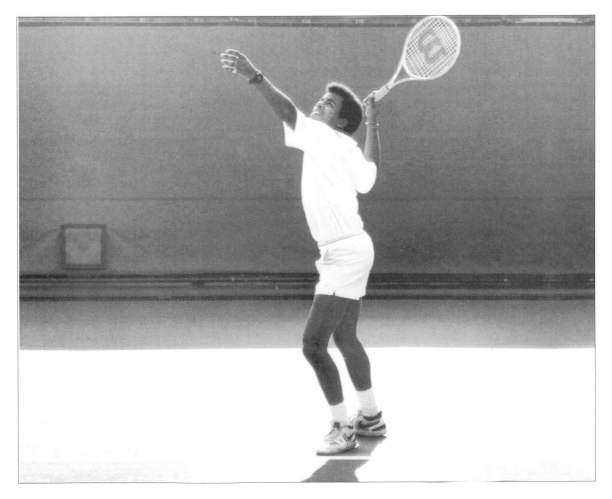

Outline

On a scale of one to ten, the importance of your serve would rate a fifteen. No other single stroke in the game of tennis gives you so many advantages, so much control of the game, and so many opportunities to score points. If you develop a good service, chances are you will develop a good, winning game. Consider the advantages of a good serve:

- You have total control of the ball. You are acting upon your opponent's game, not reacting to it.
- You have the psychological advantage of being on the attack, putting your opponent on the defensive.
- You can win points without tiresome running, chasing, and wearing yourself out.
- You can compensate for weakness in the rest of your game.

Conversely, consider the disadvantages of not developing your serve:

- You can lose points and games faster with a bad serve than with any other underdeveloped stroke—by double-faulting.
- You can lose points and games by giving your opponent easy setups and returns that can be "put away" for points.
- You can become discouraged, throwing off the rest of your game.

The Grip

There are two grips for the serve: the standard eastern forehand grip and the modified backhand grip, called the continental. The eastern forehand grip gives you a fast, bullet-type serve. Some players use it only on the first serve, while others use it for both first and second. The continental grip sacrifices speed but gives you more spin and more control of the ball. A great many players use this grip for both serves to gain accurate placement of the ball and to give the ball that spin that throws off an opponent's attempted return.

The Stance

You should serve from near the middle of the court you are defending. This means that if you are serving in a singles match, you will generally stand within 2 feet of the center of the singles court. In a doubles match, you will serve from a wider position, because you will have to defend the alley on your side of the court.

If you don't stand correctly, you can't serve correctly. In singles, to serve to your opponent's forehand court, stand behind the baseline and 1 or 2 feet to the right of the center line. This position is best for placing shallow, angled serves that go out of court before your opponent can reach them or that hit exactly on or near the service center line. If you want to serve wider, just move farther away from the center line. So if you want to force your opponent to play a wide backhand return from the ad (left) court, move a few feet farther to the left before you serve.

When you take your stance, put your left foot about an inch behind the baseline and at a 45-degree angle so that your toes point toward the net post to your right. Your right foot should be about shoulder width from your left and about parallel to the baseline. An imaginary line from your right big toe to your left big toe, if extended, will show you where the ball will land in the service court.

When your feet are in position, shift your weight to your front foot. Take a look at the court to which you are serving. Bounce the ball two, three, or four times, while breathing deeply, relaxing, and concentrating on the serve. This bouncing helps you start the rhythm so important to a good serve. Stretch your right arm and racket back. When you're ready to start your serve, shift your weight back to your right leg and go into your ready position.

Ready Position

Your forward leg should be slightly flexed, the back leg flexed just a bit more. You should have more weight on your rear leg. Lean your body out a little to the right as you point the top of your racket at your opponent. Your left hand not only holds the ball you're going to serve but cradles the racket at the throat. Remember, you're now into the rhythm of your serving action, so don't stay in the ready position very long. Look again at the spot where you are going to serve, and fix it in your mind.

The ready position
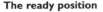
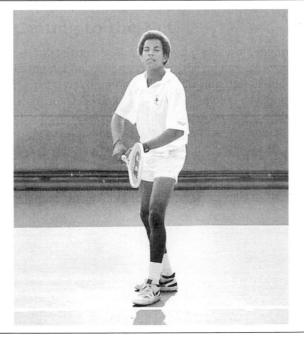

Four-Count System for Serves

Count One: The Backswing and Toss

For a good, strong backswing, both arms must go down together and come up together. Drop your left arm a bit, and then move it up in front of you and to the right. At the same time, drop the racket down behind you and to the right.

Start both arms upward at the same moment, moving your left shoulder forward and to the right. At exactly the same moment, shift weight to the front leg, bending that front knee a little. (It's important not to pick your left foot off the ground because you're going to have to pivot on it.)

The *toss* is probably the most important part of the serving action. Hold the ball you're going to serve on the fingertips of your left hand. As the left hand reaches shoulder height, toss or "push" the ball straight up—without spin. The correct height for your toss is a point where the middle of your strings can meet the ball when your right arm is fully extended upward. At that spot, the ball will be motionless when you hit it, so your chances of error are less. If the toss is too low you will be jammed and not be able to extend your arm. Tossing the ball too high is the worst thing you can do for your timing. You will have to stop everything and wait for it to come down, then hit it.

**Count One:
The backswing and
toss**

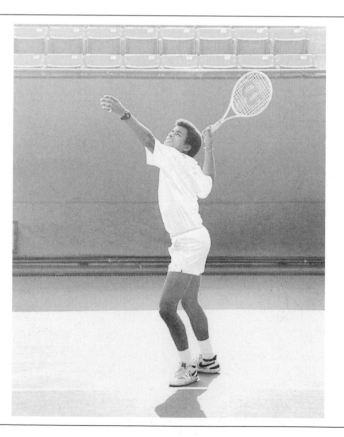

You can practice the height of your toss by holding your racket straight up against a tennis court fence and noting where the center of the racket comes. Then try tossing the ball to hit that spot again and again and again. You also want to toss the ball in such a way that if it fell, it would land a few inches in front of your front foot.

If your toss is too far forward, you may be hitting into the net, because your racket head will already be heading down in your follow-through. If your toss is too far back, you will tend to hit long, because your racket will still be heading upward when it contacts the ball.

Keep your head up and your eyes on the ball, until you finish. After releasing the ball, your hand should stay facing the sky, palm up and pointing to the ball. Remember, as mentioned earlier, the right arm not only goes down but also comes up with the left arm. When you take your left arm down to start the toss, drop your right arm, putting the racket head below your wrist and close to the ground so you can get a pendulum effect on your upswing. When your left arm lifts, bring the right one up, bending it at the elbow when the racket head gets above your shoulder. The correct position here forms a V, with the left arm in front of you, the right arm behind you, and both above your head.

Count Two: The Elbow Bend

This count is the most important part of your serve. When you get both arms up and are ready to hit the ball, move your right elbow forward and up, ahead of your arm and toward the net. This bends your arm back toward your shoulders and puts your forearm next to your biceps. It also cocks your wrist. You need both the whipping action from your elbow plus the snapping action of your wrist to get a good, point-winning serve.

The action is very much like throwing a ball. You shift your weight forward, your hips will turn toward the net, your shoulders will turn, and your elbow will straighten—and then your wrist will supply power. The sequence is just like throwing. The difference is that, in throwing, your elbow will be at shoulder height and your wrist just above your head. But in the tennis serve, your elbow and wrist will be as high over your head as you can reach.

If your wrist is relaxed as your elbow starts forward, the racket head will nearly touch your lower back. It is only from here that you can get the powerful whipping action in your serve. Only now are you ready to go after the ball with the racket.

Count Three: Making Contact with the Ball

Be sure your head stays up all the way through contact with the ball. You can't hit what you can't see. On the first serve, time your contact so that the racket will meet the ball at its highest point, before it starts dropping. If it drops, it will hit low on your racket and go into the net. On the second serve, however, you can let the ball drop an inch or two because you want to get more spin on the ball. When you

Count Two:
The elbow bend

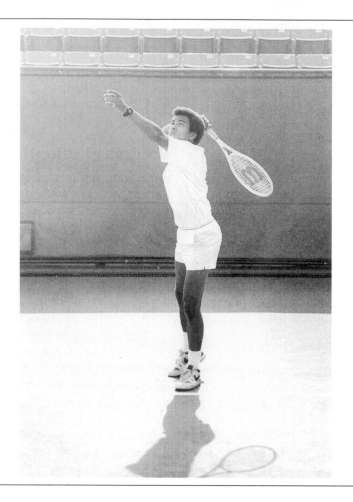

hit the ball, use all of that behind-the-back wind-up for whipping action and then, just before making contact, snap your wrist up and through the ball.

The rhythm on this stroke is important. Start your backswing slowly, move your arm up and, with a relaxed wrist, drop the racket head behind your back; then whip rapidly up and through the hit, without pausing anywhere from start to finish. Some players whisper to themselves, "S-l-o-w, FAST!" as they go through the serving action.

There are two more body movements during the hit. Your left arm will come down naturally as the racket is going up to meet the ball. Your right leg comes forward because your hip is turning toward the net. Since you are leaning forward on your left leg, your right leg will step forward, and you will catch your balance on it after you have hit the ball. If you are going to follow your serve to the net, your right leg follow-through will give you your first step toward the net. If desired, you can land on your left leg first and then step quickly forward with your right leg (for right-handers).

**Count Three:
Making contact with
the ball**

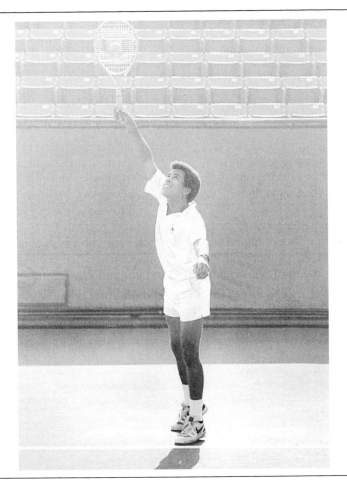

Count Four: The Follow-Through

Make sure your head is still up and your eyes are on the ball. After the racket hits the ball, keep it moving in the desired direction for a few inches, then bring the racket down your right side before crossing your body and finishing at the left. The whipping action of your elbow and the snap of your wrist should have the racket head speeding along by now, so make sure you don't perform open leg surgery with it.

In addition to the whip and snap, you also need your entire body behind the serve. If you put everything into your serve, your weight will be completely over your forward leg, and your hips will be turned toward the net. This will bring your rear leg forward naturally. As your rear leg steps forward into the court, you will regain your balance. And if you decide to follow your serve to the net to attack your opponent, you will have already taken your first step toward the net.

Count Four:
The follow-through

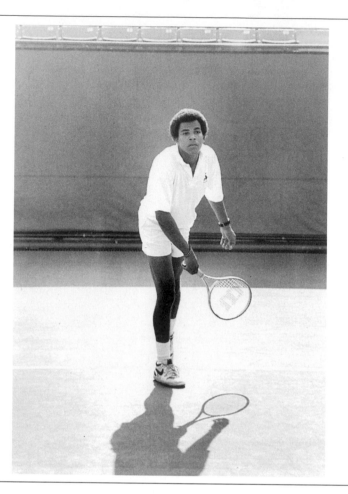

| ✓ | *Checklist for Serves—Right-Handed Players* |

1. Be sure to get a good rhythm just before starting the ball toss.
2. Learn how to make a perfect ball toss, and keep your left arm up after the toss.
3. Get a good knee bend and shoulder turn (coiled position) just before contact.
4. Get fast racket-head speed by using your elbow in a throwing motion and snapping your wrist.
5. Follow through quickly with a couple of steps into the court.

Full sequence for the serve—right-handed player

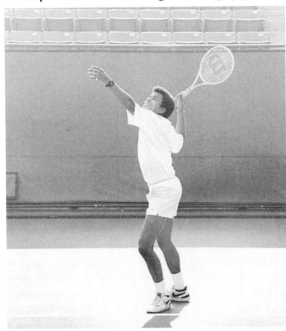

Count One: The backswing and toss

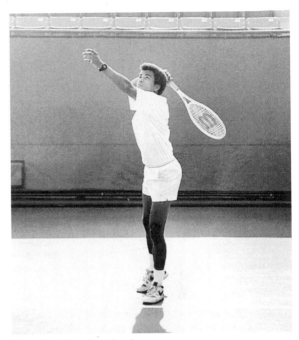

Count Two: The elbow bend

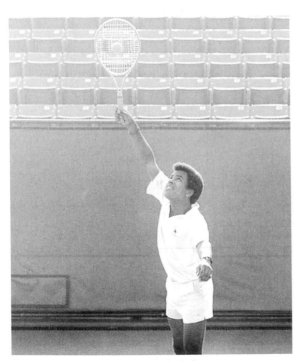

Count Three: Making contact with the ball

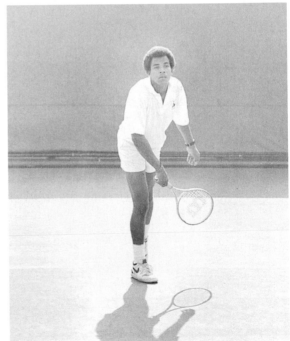

Count Four: The follow-through

Full sequence for the serve—left-handed player

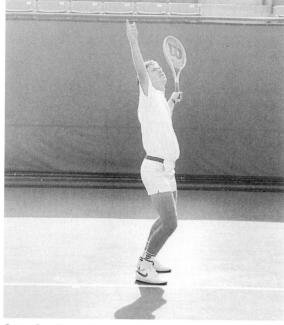

Count One: The backswing and toss

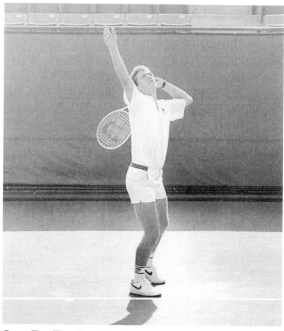

Count Two: The elbow bend

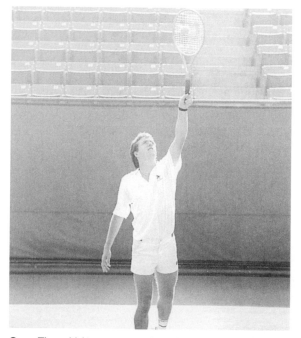

Count Three: Making contact with the ball

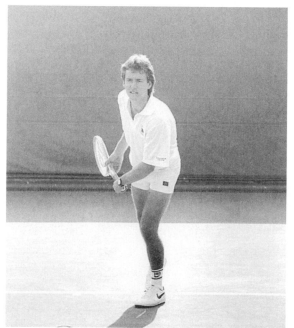

Count Four: The follow-through

✓	*Checklist for Serves—Left-Handed Players*

1. Be sure to get a good rhythm just before starting the ball toss.
2. Learn how to make a perfect ball toss, and keep your right arm up after the toss.
3. Get a good knee bend and shoulder turn (coiled position) just before contact.
4. Get fast racket-head speed by using your elbow in a throwing motion and snapping your wrist.
5. Follow through quickly with a couple of steps into the court.

The Rhythm of the Serve

The serve has a definite rhythm to it, with different parts of your body working smoothly to create the overall stroke. Learning that rhythm, especially where it speeds up, is absolutely essential to a good serve. Remember, Count One starts off slowly, and then Two, Three, and Four speed up: 1—2-3-4 fast! Never stop or pause between counts. You're trying to develop one continuous motion from the backswing until the completion of the follow-through.

Types of Serves

There are three kinds of serves you should learn. Each is used for a different type of situation, opponent, or game. Most good players mix them up.

Flat Serve

The flat serve is a power serve with no spin. It travels in a straight line. It can make a strong first serve because you hit the racket flat through the ball. It is usually a low-percentage serve, and if it's not working for you, abandon it. However, if it's going in and earning points, stay with it until it weakens, then switch to another serve.

One psychological disadvantage of the fast, hard, flat serve is that when it does go in, you expect either a weak return or none at all. Should the return come back to you just as fast as you sent it, you're likely to be unable to move from the back court quickly enough to return it. Its main advantage is a speed that can leave slower opponents just standing there watching you "ace" them.

Beginners will usually start out by using a soft flat serve because it is easy to learn. The soft serve will not keep a good opponent off balance, however. A hard flat serve will. It takes an expert to hit a hard flat serve, though, because the margin of error is so small. The spin serves give a much greater margin of error.

The flat serve—right- and left-handed player

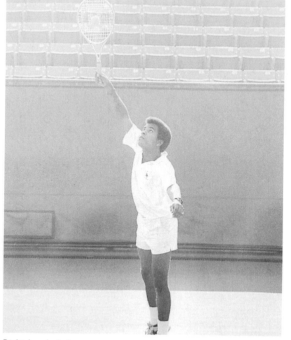

Right-handed player   Left-handed player

Slice

After learning the basic flat-serving motion, the beginner can work on the slice, which is a much more effective serve. The spin of this serve allows you to serve higher over the net but still have the ball come down in the service court.

The slice is a left-hander's dream because it "slices" the ball to the backhand side of the opponent in both courts. If you are a southpaw, use it most of the time. For right-handers, this service is best when serving to the forehand court, because it can slice off to your opponent's right and out of the court after it bounces, or it can squeeze the right-handed receiver when returning the backhand. The major disadvantage is that it is difficult to place the slice into the right-handed receiver's backhand, because the receiver can run around it for a forehand return. The slice is also a strong, effective serve when sent to a left-hander, because it goes easily to the backhand and away from the receiver.

To slice the serve, move your body around faster than for the flat serve. Toss the ball more in front of you and more to the right. Hit the ball on its right half, and make sure the racket stays with the ball until it gives a good slice action. A well-hit slice should curve to the left when it leaves your racket and continue curving to the left as it kicks off its bounce.

The slice serve—right- and left-handed player

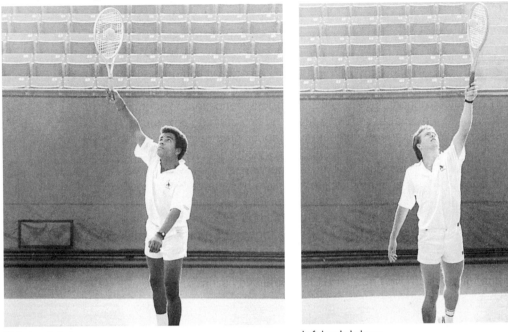

Right-handed player   Left-handed player

Topspin

The topspin is the best all-around serve for a right-hander, because it is controllable and fast; also, it has variations and is easy to hit into a right-hander's backhand. The topspin serve is hard to return because it's unpredictable, bouncing straight back or to the receiver's left after it hits.

To put topspin on the ball, hit it under the left side and peel your racket up and through the top right side in a left-to-right racket motion. On the first serve, toss the ball a little more to the left and a little more in front of you, and don't put too much spin on it. If that doesn't give the desired effect, then add more spin, or go to variations for your second serve.

This serve should be learned early. In fact, your second serve should be learned before your first serve so that you have confidence in always getting your serve in.

Serving Strategy

A good serve is 50 percent fundamentals and 50 percent knowing what to do with it—the placement, the speed, the spin. The serve should be a high percentage shot. You should reach the stage where the great majority of your first

The topspin serve—right- and left-handed player

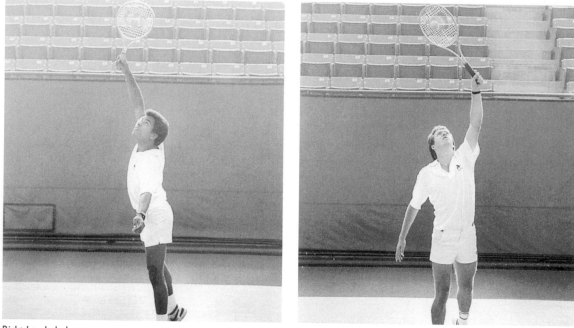

Right-handed player   Left-handed player

serves go in; and when they don't, you should be able to place your second serve into the opponent's backhand, where there is less chance of returning it.

Because most opponents expect a weaker second serve, put more power into it every now and then, catching your opponent flat-footed and unprepared to return it. However, if you are winning or getting a good percentage of your serves in, don't change what you are doing. Stay with it until the percentages turn against you.

Use a change of pace on the placement and speed of your serves. Don't serve to the same place with the same speed all the time. Keep your opponent guessing. Mix up serves to forehands and backhands, slow and fast serves, flats, spins, and slices.

Remember, you're serving to the court, not to the opponent. If you watch the other player, his or her moves and shifts may confuse you and cause double-faults. Instead, look at the spot on the court where you want the ball to go, and serve there. Don't let your opponent's hops, jumps, skips, and lunges fool you into serving up exactly the ball he or she can put away.

Serve to your opponent's weakness on the big points. Also, serve the ball right at your opponent every once in a while (especially on first serves). This is called the jam serve.

Summary

1. The serve is just another 1-2-3-4 action—but it is the most important one.

2. Your serve must be consistent. The service break, where you win a game when your opponent is serving, is what usually wins a match. So you can't let your opponent break your serve if you want to win matches.

3. As you serve, observe the following guidelines:
   - Your weight should shift to your rear foot as you get into the ready position.
   - Your weight should shift forward as the racket starts forward and up. The toss should begin as your racket starts upward.
   - The toss should be exactly as high as the middle of the racket head when it is extended over your head.
   - Your elbow should straighten, and your wrist should snap the racket up and through the ball.
   - Your rear leg will come forward naturally as you lean into your serve.

4. Most beginners learn a soft flat serve first but soon come to rely on the slice serve. Advanced players use the slice, topspin, and hard flat serves.

Drills for the Beginner

1. *The Toss Height.* Standing next to a fence or wall, reach as high as possible with your racket. If possible, mark the spot of the top of your racket. Now toss the ball to that spot. A perfect toss would be exactly at the middle of your racket (the sweet spot) at the top of its arc. By tossing to the top of your racket, you allow yourself a small margin of error.

2. *Placing the Toss.* Take your serving stance, and place your racket on the ground with the head just ahead of and to the net side of your forward foot. Toss the ball to the proper height and let it drop to the ground. If it hits your racket head, it is placed perfectly.

3. *Serving into a Fence* allows you to perfect the serving action without worrying about whether or not the ball will go into the service court.

4. *Serving from the Service Line* gives you a much easier target to hit. Just stand at the service line, and serve to the opposite service court.

Drill for Intermediate and Advanced Players

This drill is discussed further and illustrated in Chapter 14.

Serving at Targets. Place targets (tennis ball cans or cardboard) on the serving court. One target should be 6 feet short of the service line and along the boundary toward which you will aim your slice serve. (For right-handed servers, it will be to the left of the court as you face it.) A second target should be in the opposite corner of the service court. (For right-handed servers, it will be to your right in the service court—that is, toward your right-handed opponent's backhand.) The third target should be exactly where your opponent will stand. (For a right-handed opponent, it will be 3 to 4 feet in from the center line and just inside the service line.)

Practice serving at each target. You will get a thrill each time you knock over a ball can with a perfect serve.

7 *Return of Service*

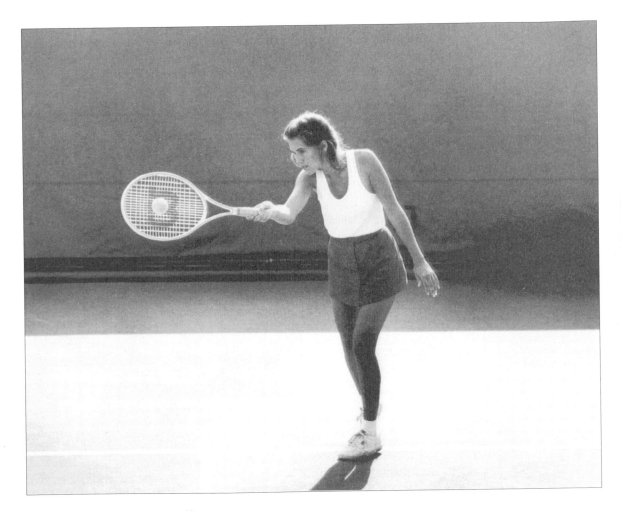

Outline

The service return is probably the most neglected shot in tennis, yet it is one of the most important. If you can't return serves, you will never break your opponent's serve, and, therefore, you will never win. It is a shot that the professionals practice frequently.

When a player returns the serve well, the opponent becomes psychologically flustered. Most players who have their serve "go out" on them have the rest of their game "go out" on them too. So the return of the serve makes these players start thinking, "What's wrong with my serve?" And they worry about it so much that their entire game deteriorates. They don't give you credit for returning the serve well; they just think that they are doing something wrong. Often their forehand or their volley or their backhand ground strokes start to falter as well—just because they have become discouraged with their serve.

Four-Count System for Forehand Return

Count One: Getting to the Ball

As soon as the server starts to throw the ball up, you must watch that ball, even though the server has not yet hit it. You must start getting up on your toes and inching forward a little bit. At this time your head is in front of your body, your shoulders are leaning forward—not off balance, but definitely leaning forward. You are moving your feet now. You should jump up a little bit off the ground and move slightly forward with "quick feet" when your opponent actually throws the ball up. You want to be attacking before your opponent has even hit the serve.

Count One:
Getting to the ball

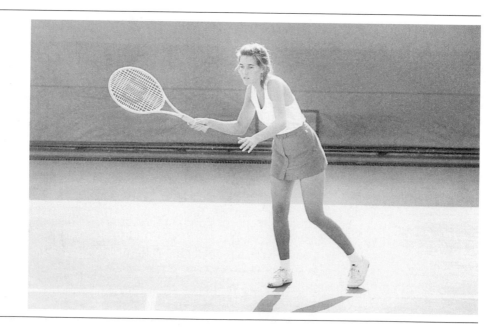

When your opponent hits the serve, you must feel as though you are going out to the ball enough so that you can hit the ball shoulder or chest high. That is the spot you want. You want this spot in order to hit that ball out and down at your opponent's feet. This way you don't have to lift the ball up over the net, and you will get the ball back more quickly. Don't let the ball start down; get the ball on the rise.

Keep your eyes on the ball. As soon as you see the ball coming off the racket, get your racket up and back, so that you will be ready to hit the ball. Then start moving your feet toward the ball. You will be moving with the racket ready. Keep your left hand out pointing at the ball. Your eyes should be level to the ball in this position.

Count Two: The Step

You want to get the ball back to your opponent before he or she gets in position to volley. This rushes your opponent. It is very much like the volley. You have to go out and intercept it. In order to hit the ball at the proper spot, you sometimes have to hurry up and meet the ball. You have to get up to it quickly.

When you have time, get set, just as you do in a forehand or backhand, with your body sideways to the net. (Right-handers will have their left foot forward on the forehand and the right foot forward on the backhand.)

Count Three: Making Contact with the Ball

Step out and hit the ball with a stroke about parallel to the ground. By hitting the ball at a high point, you do not have to hit it up and over the net. Keep your

**Count Two:
The step**

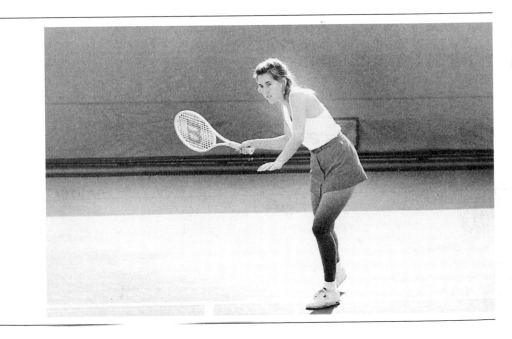

**Count Three:
Making contact with
the ball**

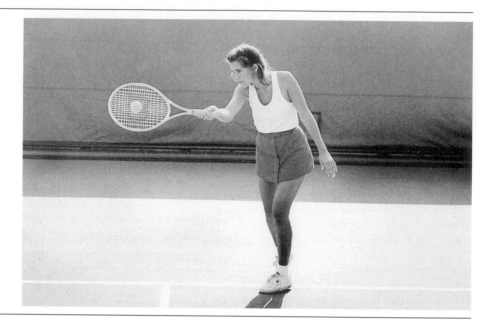

head level all the time. You do not lift your head up at any time as you might have to do on a regular ground stroke. During all of this time, you are going out to meet the ball. The hit is not under the ball—it is right through the ball.

The intermediate player can add a bit of finesse by bringing the racket over the ball and applying topspin as it is hit.

When your opponent is hitting hard first serves, don't swing at them; just block them. Use a short backswing and a short follow-through. You block the ball this way when you don't have enough time to hit a full shot.

Your opponent's second serve will probably be hit more softly. Therefore, move in on the baseline, even inside the baseline, and swing at the ball a little harder. Try to get a little more power into your return, and try to hit the ball when it is shoulder high as you did on the first serve.

Never slice your forehand return of serve. Always hit it flat or with a little bit of topspin. Only in a very rare instance, when you're in a lot of trouble and reaching way out to your right, should you consider slicing the forehand return of serve. Otherwise, either hit it flat or use topspin.

Use whichever serve return is working for you on a given day. If you are not hitting the slice well some days, then you should be able to drive, and vice versa; consequently, it is important to perfect your skills in both. If your opponent's second serve has a big spin, you should probably try to slice the ball, because it is a little easier to slice than to drive when you are hitting high-bouncing balls.

**Count Four:
The follow-through**

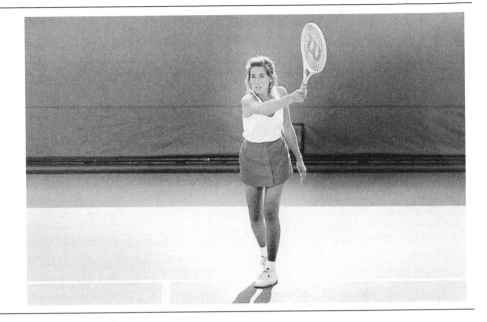

Count Four: The Follow-Through

The follow-through is absolutely essential. You lock into your follow-through position with your right arm up against your left shoulder as you did on the regular ground stroke. Do not follow through very far, especially on the first serve, where you want to just block it. On the second serve, though, you can follow through a little farther. Continue through the ball after you hit it. Then move to the position you want on the court.

✓	*Checklist for Service Return*

1. Get up on your toes just before the service action.
2. Use your eyes. Watch the ball from the point when your opponent starts the service toss.
3. Move forward to return the ball just as it is starting to rise from its bounce in the service court.
4. Take a short backswing—especially on the first serve.
5. On a second serve, move closer to the net.
6. Concentrate on the ball.
7. If you return well, your opponent will lose confidence and not serve well.

Four-Count System for Backhand Return

Count One: Getting to the Ball

Pick your racket up, and start moving to the ball. Your racket should be up in the same position for both the slice and the drive, since you are going to be hitting the ball about shoulder high. Your opponent will not know which return you are going to use—the slice or the drive. Your head is forward. Your body is forward. And you are moving to the ball and still facing the net a bit.

Count Two: The Step

As you shift your weight to your front (right) leg, your body should turn a little sideways toward the net. At this point, you are about ready to hit. Your eyes are level to the ball. If you do not have time to get in this position, you will have to hit with your weight on your rear foot, which is difficult.

When your opponent hits the serve, step out with your right leg and make the return. You will hit off your right leg and push forward from it. For your backhand, you should step out with your outside leg (left leg), then cross over onto your front leg (right leg). Do this on both a slice and a topspin shot. After the hit, hop forward on the right leg if you want an offensive shot.

Count Three: Making Contact with the Ball

You hit the ball off your front leg if possible. The ball should be about a foot in front of your front leg. You are hitting the ball with a stroke about parallel to the ground if you are hitting a drive.

On your backhand return, you should be able to slice or drive the ball. Be able to do both well. A sliced return of serve is usually a very safe shot. It should be low and close to the opponent's feet. And try to get the ball back quickly, before the server is set. You can drive it or put topspin on it—either is very effective as an offensive return.

Count Four: The Follow-Through

If you are returning a first serve, you should not follow through too far. On a second serve, however, you follow through a little farther to get more power. Continue on through the shot, then return to a good attacking or defending position back on the court.

If you are an intermediate or advanced player, you will want to follow through over the top of the ball just a little so that you can hit it down at your opponent's feet. Or if you slice, the bottom edge should lead a little to get the proper amount of spin. But don't let your bottom edge lead too much, or you'll have too much spin and not enough power. Be sure to complete a strong follow-through.

The forehand return—the full sequence

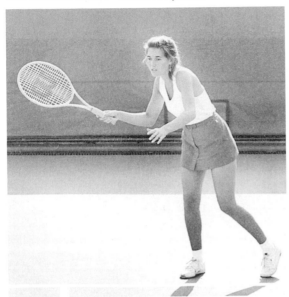

Count One: Getting to the ball

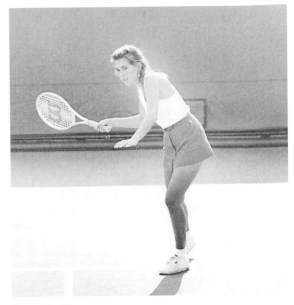

Count Two: The step

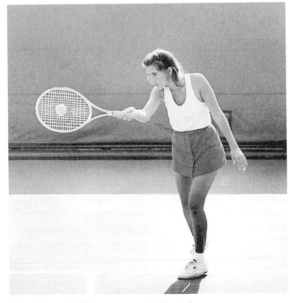

Count Three: Making contact with the ball

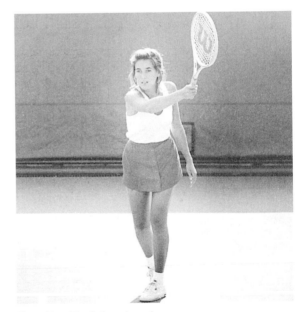

Count Four: The follow-through

The Backhand—the full sequence

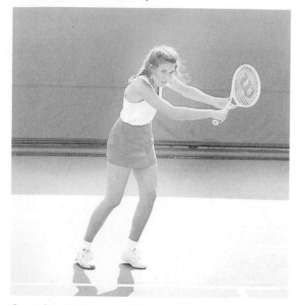

Count One: Getting to the ball

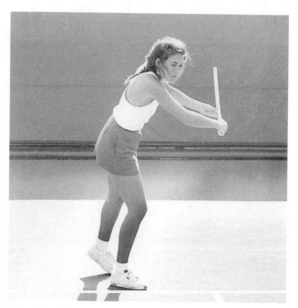

Count Two: The step

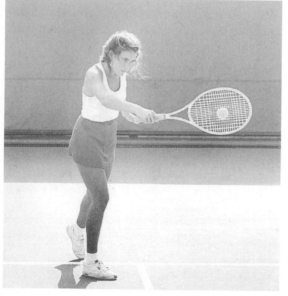

Count Three: Making contact with the ball

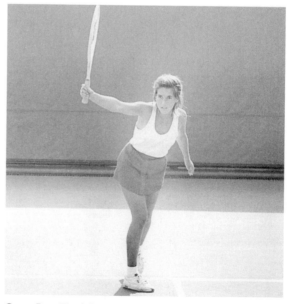

Count Four: The follow-through

Service Return Strategy

You can't let your opponent rush you if you are not ready to return the serve. Just keep your head down until you are ready to make the return shot. Don't let the server force you to either wait or be rushed by him or her.

For the first serve, you will usually stand about 3 feet behind the baseline, halfway between where your opponent might serve to your forehand or your backhand. You should not leave any open space.

If your opponent serves mostly to your forehand, you should move a little bit to the right. If he or she serves to your backhand most of the time, you should move a little bit to the left. Most good players will mix it up. They will serve some to your forehand and some to your backhand. So you have to be halfway between.

Don't always stand in the same place. Instead of standing 3 feet behind the baseline for the first serve, sometimes stand on the baseline or 6 or 8 feet in back of the baseline. Don't always give the server the same perspective. Move around a little bit: up and back, left and right. If you stand in the same place all the time and hit the same return, the ball is always going to get back to the server at the same time, and the server will come to know when to make the volley. You must change pace (ball speed) and change your position a little bit so that your opponent will be hitting the ball in a different place every time.

When you are starting a match, don't try to produce winning shots. You are nervous, and so is your opponent. Just keep the ball in play. Make your opponent hit a few volleys. Also, don't try to hit for the sidelines at the start of the match. Hit more down the middle, because if you hit poorly, which is common, the ball is more likely to stay in bounds.

Early in the match, try to return the serve by just blocking the ball and hitting it at your opponent's feet. You don't have much time to do anything else, unless you are playing very well. Get it back quickly before your opponent has time to get set.

If the server stays back, there's no need for you to do very much with a return serve. All you need to do is hit it as a regular ground stroke. You should get a little bit farther back behind the baseline than you normally would so that the ball will peak over and come down just as a regular ground stroke. You hit this shot deep with no pressure at all because you know that the server is not coming to the net.

The main thing is not to miss this type of return, because if you get it back fairly deep in the court, you have neutralized the other person's serving advantage. Don't try to do too much with this shot. If you can hit the ball back to your opponent's backhand, that's even better. What you do not want to do is hit very short so your opponent can approach on the next shot or put it away on you.

If you have a server who comes into the net but who has a weak volley, you should still return the serve as a regular ground stroke. Don't try to do too much. Don't rush it. Just hit a normal ground stroke. This type of server is probably coming to the net just to intimidate you, hoping that you will miss. But you must get the ball back in play and force a volley. Your opponent might hit a few volleys away for points, which might frighten you into trying to make better returns. But if you just keep returning the ball steadily and consistently, your opponent's weak volley will show up. Don't play in a hit-and-miss fashion. Make your opponent volley. Keep hitting regular ground strokes. Keep your eye on the ball, and don't watch the server come in.

Usually, the second serve is hit more gently than the first but with more spin. The slice serve will bounce low. The topspin will bounce very high. So you have to move up to it to get to the ball before it spins away or bounces too high to hit effectively.

Sometimes you can't move in at all if the second serve is very strong. But most of the time it isn't, so you can come inside the baseline. When you move in closer, let your opponent see you move in so as to add a little pressure to the situation. Even if you do not intend to play from that point, let your opponent see you move in, then move back before he serves.

Also, on the second serve it's often a good idea to move over a little to your left and run around your backhand to hit your forehand return of the serve. It's better to hit with your forehand even if you have a better backhand, because when your opponent is serving and volleying it's very difficult for him or her to read a forehand return of serve. It is easier to volley the backhand return of serve.

You must let your opponent see you move to your left as though you are going to run around and hit your forehand. Sometimes the server will try to change serves in mid-swing to take advantage of what you are doing. But such a change of strategy can lead to a double-fault or a poor serve. So try to out-smart and pressure the server—make him or her wonder what you are going to do—but don't miss returning the serve. If you start missing returns, you are going to take the pressure off the server.

With the second serve you have more time to swing at the ball and try to go for a winner more often, either down to the opponent's backhand or over to his or her forehand. You can hurt your opponent more on second serves. Every once in a while, make an offensive shot on the second serve; that is, attack the ball as you would an approach shot. Come into the net, and try to take it away from your opponent. This will surprise and pressure the server.

A type of return of serve you never see that should be used more often is the lob. This return forces your opponent, who is rushing the net, to make an overhead shot. And sometimes the overhead is hard to hit while coming in very fast. An opponent may be so used to hitting volleys that he or she is not ready to hit an overhead.

Summary

1. The return of service is an absolutely essential part of the game. Since your opponent's strongest weapon should be the serve, you must be able to neutralize it with your return. In this way, you take away your opponent's advantage and cause the rally to become even.

2. You must start for the ball as it leaves your opponent's racket.
   - You will need only a short backswing.
   - Block the ball if it is hard hit.
   - Follow through with topspin to help bring it down in bounds.
3. Keep your opponent off balance by changing the place where you assume your ready position. Sometimes be up, sometimes back, sometimes right, sometimes left.
4. Your major objective should be to get the ball in play.

Drills for Players at All Levels

These drills are further discussed and illustrated in Chapter 14.

1. *Service return.* Have a partner stand close to the service line of the opposite court and serve you the ball. By being closer, your partner has a better chance of getting the ball in the court, and you will have to react faster to make your shot.
2. *Serve and return* allows the players to practice the two most difficult aspects of the game.

8 *Approach Shots*

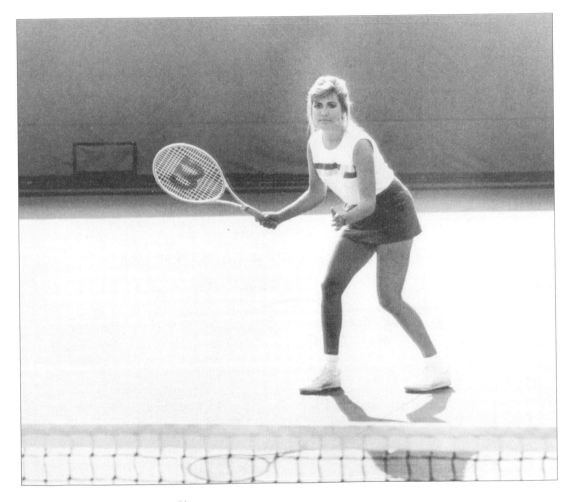

Outline

The approach shot is used as you come to the net to attack your opponent. It is played differently in technique and in strategy than other shots, and it is important to learn these differences.

You will generally decide to go to the net when you have the advantage. (Your advantage can come when you have made a strong serve or return or when your opponent has made a weak short return.) You usually hit your approach shot while you are running forward. Your racket should contact the ball at a height somewhere between your waist and your shoulders, considerably higher than most ground strokes. Hitting it there gives you two advantages: your chances of putting the ball into the net are slim, and you get the ball back to your opponent faster, with the chance of rushing him or her into making a mistake.

On forehand approach shots, hit the ball hard and fairly flat for depth, adding a touch of topspin for control. If you are scooping up a low ball, add more topspin to lift it over the net.

The backhand approach shot is different. Here, especially when you are running hard to the ball, the slice becomes your best shot. The only exception might be if you are meeting the ball at a height above the net; then you should drive it flat. Otherwise, the backhand slice helps you get the shot off faster, and it helps you get you to the net faster when hitting on the run.

Four-Count System for Approach Shots

Count One: Getting to the Ball

Start rushing up to meet the ball when you realize it is going to come in short. Get your racket into a short, high backswing instantly. Because you are going to hit the ball at a higher point than you do most shots, the racket should go back and stay back at a higher point. A long backswing will throw you off balance and slow up your run. While you are running, hold the racket with only one hand, using the other to help you keep balanced as you rush forward.

Face the ball and the net as you run toward them. Use long steps to cover ground rapidly, but as you get closer to the ball, shorten them to give yourself maximum balance. Once again, your body should be low, head in front of your feet, and eyes low and level to the ball.

Count Two: Getting Ready to Make Contact with the Ball

Get ready to hit as you get close to the ball, moving your free hand to the shaft of the racket. On the forehand, just touch the racket before taking it back farther. On the backhand, you should usually use your free hand to help complete the backswing, and do not let go until you start the racket forward to meet the ball.

Because you are running, make sure to get your racket head out ahead of your body to meet the ball before it gets to you. Don't run through the ball and hit it late. The best way to avoid this is to make sure your head and shoulders are leaning out in front of your legs and feet, your eyes level to the ball and

Count One: Getting to the ball—forehand and backhand

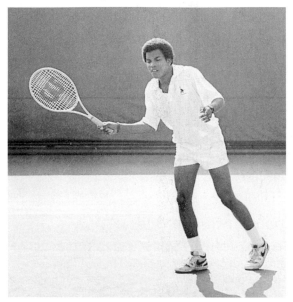

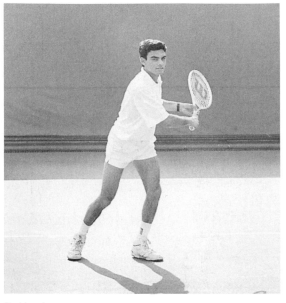

Forehand

Backhand

Count Two: Getting ready to make contact—forehand and backhand

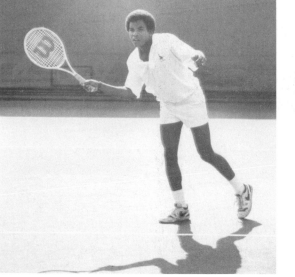

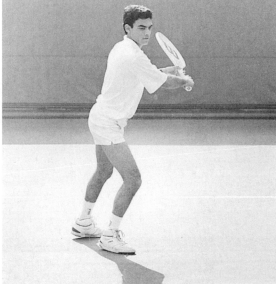

Forehand

Backhand

parallel to the ground during the entire stroke. Your swing should stay about parallel to the ground, and the racket should meet the ball above your waist, or better yet, at chest or shoulder height.

- For the forehand, make your step forward, and then push off with your right leg just before contact. This helps you run right through the ball while keeping your balance.
- For the backhand, you have two options: You can step onto your right leg, hit the ball, then hop forward on that same leg. This step seems to work for high approaches and those that you hit down the line. Or you can step forward with your left leg while you are hitting. This keeps you moving rapidly into the net. It seems to work best for low approach shots.

Practice both of these steps to find out which is the most comfortable and effective for you

Count Three: Making Contact with the Ball

As you hit, keep your racket in contact with the ball after you hit it, then follow through as if you hit a ground stroke. Also, keep your body leaning forward while you run toward the net. Do not pull up, away from the shot, and do not look to see where the ball is going. When you slice the backhand approach shot, your head and right shoulder should lean in the direction you want the ball to go.

Count Three: Making contact with the ball—forehand and backhand

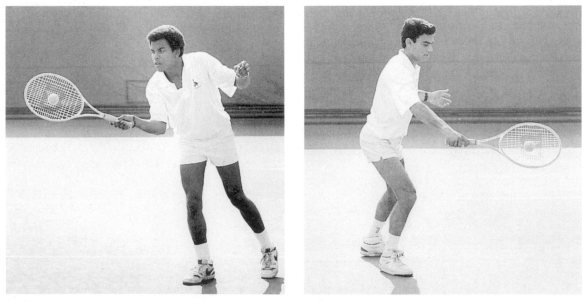

Forehand   Backhand

Count Four: The follow-through—forehand and backhand

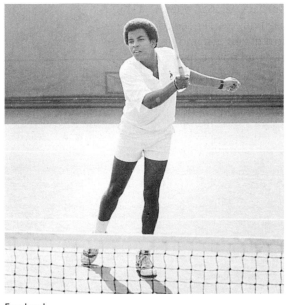

Forehand

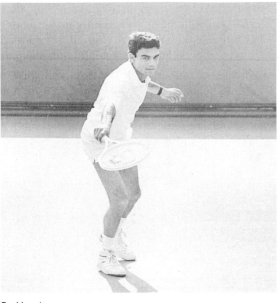

Backhand

A surprising number of approach shots can be sure put-aways if you get good depth on them. Keep trying to read your opponent to spot weaknesses, then take advantage of them. If you have spotted a weak forehand or backhand in your opponent, hit your approach shot to that side.

Generally try to hit your approach shot down the line. Sometimes you can hit down the middle. Your opponent has to take time to decide between a forehand or backhand return, and in that momentary confusion can become "hand-cuffed." Also, it is hard to get a good angle on a passing return when it comes down the middle.

You may need to vary your approach shot in two ways. You may need to change your pace (ball speed) against some players. Now and then float a slow, easy, high approach to upset your opponent's timing and perhaps psych him or her into making a mistake.

Also, changing spins may be necessary, because some players cannot handle them very well. Hit the ball with backspin, which keeps it low, or with topspin, which makes it jump erratically after it bounces.

Aim your forehand approach shots down the line most of the time—to your opponent's backhand. Your backhand approach shot can be hit either down the line to your opponent's forehand or cross-court to the backhand. A down-the-line approach has the advantage of staying low, but it has the disadvantage of going to your opponent's forehand, which is likely to be his or her strongest stroke. If you go to the cross-court return, hit it deep—deeper than the down-the-line return, so your opponent cannot step into it with maximum power and control.

If you are playing someone who moves well, don't necessarily hit your approach to the open court. Many times, you can get the point by hitting the ball behind your opponent, especially if you can catch that player on the wrong foot or going the wrong way. But if your opponent is slow, definitely place it in the open area.

The full sequence for the forehand approach shot

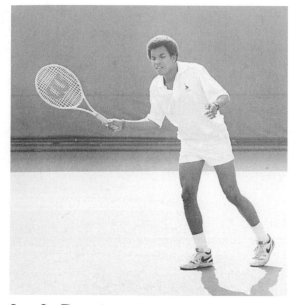

Count One: The running position

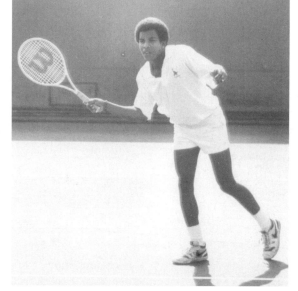

Count Two: Getting ready for contact

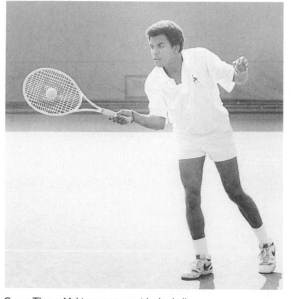

Count Three: Making contact with the ball

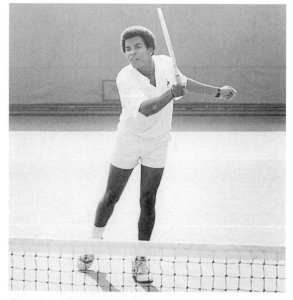

Count Four: The follow-through

Count Four: The Follow-Through

After your shot, continue running toward the net. Your steps will be different than for other ground strokes. After you hit the ball, lengthen your stride again to get to your net position fast; then get set just before your opponent tries to

The full sequence for the backhand approach shot

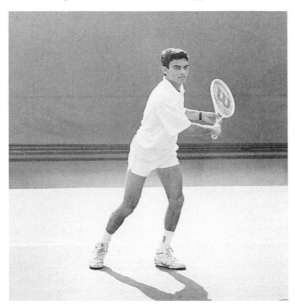

Count One: The running position

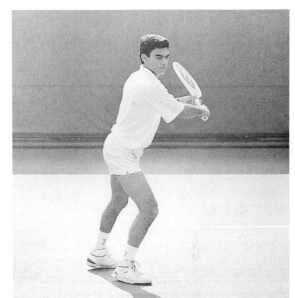

Count Two: Getting ready for contact

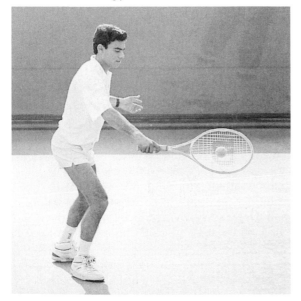

Count Three: Making contact with the ball

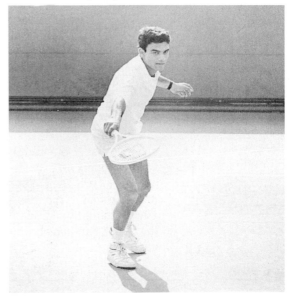

Count Four: The follow-through

> ✓ *Checklist for Approach Shots*
>
> 1. Hit the ball on the run as you continue toward the net.
> 2. Hit hard to keep your opponent on the defensive.
> 3. Hit your shots down the line unless you are going for a winner, in which case you should go cross-court.
> 4. Hit the ball at a higher point than a ground stroke so that you don't have to lift it up and over the net.

hit a passing shot. If your shot went down the middle, take the middle of the net. If it went down either side, take that side. A good volley can offset a ground stroke and give you an overall winning game.

Drop Shot

The drop shot should be hit with backspin. This makes the ball stop when it hits the ground, and is harder for your opponent to reach. Hit the ball so that it lands barely over the net; the closer the better. Clearance above the net should be low—the ball gets over the net faster, which gives less time for your opponent to react.

Don't pop the drop shot up too high above the net. This is a touch shot. When you hit the ball you should have soft hands so that you have feel. Hit the ball delicately. After contact, go through the ball a few inches to feel the backspin, then give with the shot.

Your opportunity to hit this shot comes when a slow, short ball inside the service line comes to you. The height of the ball can vary, but it is usually hit lower than the net. If a ball is hit short and high, you would probably hit an approach shot. Also, your opponent must be behind the baseline before you hit this shot.

Acting like you are going to approach and then drop-shotting can be very effective. Take your racket back like you are going to approach. This makes your opponent go back deeper into the court. Act like you are going to hit the approach hard, then at the last minute hit the drop shot. Acting is easy to do on the backhand as the drop shot is hit like your slice, with the racket hand up. Since you rarely slice the forehand, deception is more difficult on this side. Pick the racket hand up above your wrist much like on a volley in order to get good backspin.

Using the drop shot can be great, as we will discuss in the strategy section, but we have seen too many players overuse it and get in trouble. The player who uses this shot too much becomes a very lazy player who wants to end the point quickly, one way or the other. This player doesn't have the good balance or court position necessary to hit this shot. Don't let yourself get in that habit. It's better for average players to overuse this shot than advanced players, since a poor drop shot doesn't hurt them as much.

We have talked about faking out your opponent, doing some "acting." Don't fake so much on any shot that you fake yourself out.

Strategy

There are two places you can hit the drop shot. One is down the line and the other is cross-court. Down the line is better to hit when you want the ball to get over the net fast. This ball does not have as far to travel to get over the net as the cross-court ball. However, your opponent doesn't have as far to run to get to the ball. Therefore, you must hit the shot well or your opponent will run it down and have an easy shot.

Down the line is easier to hit as the ball doesn't have far to go. You just block this shot instead of trying to get the racket head around to angle the ball cross-court. This shot must land closer to the net than the cross-court, since it is hit in the direction of your opponent rather than away.

Hitting cross-court is very effective in pulling your opponent out of court so that you can put away the return. Even though this shot has farther to travel to its destination than down the line, your opponent has further to run and so must run up and out of court. The angled (cross-court) shot is probably better against a fast player, because it is a good way to get your opponent out of court for the next shot. This might be the safer shot as your ball doesn't have to land so close to the net. The down-the-line should be better against a slower opponent.

Opponents who reach a well-hit down-the-line drop shot are coming closer and closer to the net and are vulnerable to a lob. Opponents who reach a well-hit cross-court drop shot are vulnerable to a ground stroke or volley to the open court.

Most opponents will see the ball coming to them better on the cross-court shot as it comes off your racket to their left or right. The down-the-line ball, however, comes more directly at them; it is hard for players to get their depth perception going fast enough to tell if the ball is short or deep. Your opponent will, therefore, get a late start to the ball.

Use this shot against a steady player who prefers ground strokes over volleys. This type of player is very difficult to play. Wait patiently until your opponent hits a short ball, and then you can hit either an approach shot or a drop shot. Mix these two up. When you use the drop shot, you will bring your opponents up to the net in unfamiliar territory where they feel uncomfortable and unsure of themselves. If you don't learn how and when to hit the drop shot, a steady player will just stay back and give you a bit of trouble.

Most players run to their left or right well, but run up and back poorly. This is because they don't have to run up and back very much and it comes as a surprise to them. As mentioned before, a player's depth perception doesn't allow him or her to judge if a ball is short or deep immediately. A player will

Full sequence for the forehand drop shot

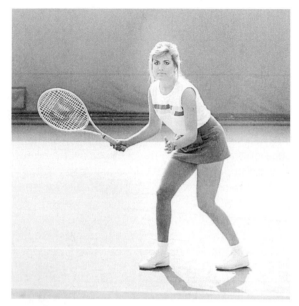

Count One: The running position

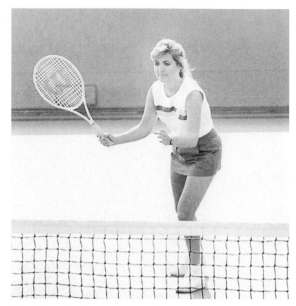

Count Two: Getting ready to make contact

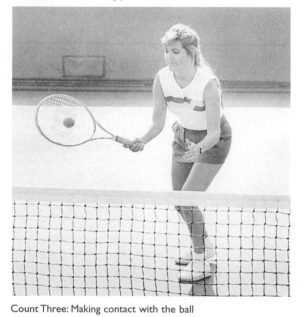

Count Three: Making contact with the ball

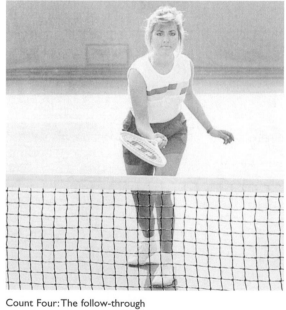

Count Four: The follow-through

hesitate before reading deep or short and, therefore, get a poor "jump" on the ball. When you hit the down-the-line drop shot, most of your opponents will have this depth perception problem.

Full sequence for the backhand drop shot

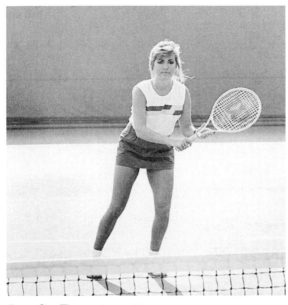

Count One: The running position

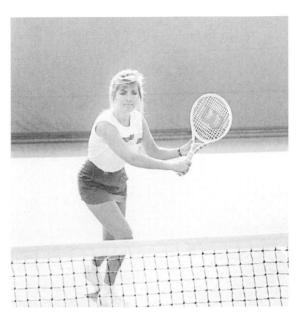

Count Two: Getting ready to make contact

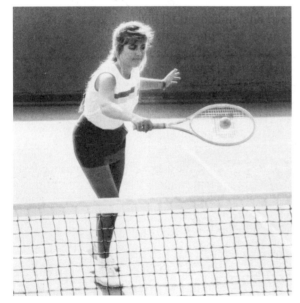

Count Three: Making contact with the ball

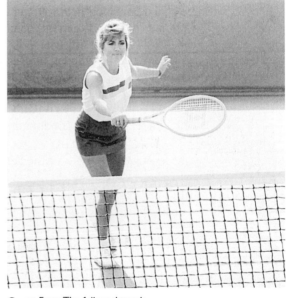

Count Four: The follow-through

Summary

1. Once you have decided to attack your opponent by playing the net, you will usually need to make one shot in midcourt as you approach the net.
2. Start running for the net as soon as you have made a strong serve or as soon as you realize that your opponent's return will be short.
3. Keep your backswing short.
4. Contact the ball at a point about chest high.
5. You will generally want to hit your forehand approach shot flat or with top spin, but you will want to slice your backhand.
6. You should usually place your shot down the line, to your opponent's weakness, or behind your opponent if he or she is running.
7. Be ready to change the speed and the spin on your approach shots—especially if you come to the net often.
8. After you have hit your shot, continue toward the net.

Drills for Players at All Levels

1. With a partner on the other side of the net, have your partner throw (for beginners) or hit a shot that lands near the service line. Approach the shot and hit it down the line or cross-court while continuing to the net.
2. During a rally, charge every short shot; make your approach shot and continue toward the net.
3. With both players at the net, let the ball bounce once on your side, then hit it just over the net, easy, low, and with backspin. Hit it down the line or cross-court, but it must be just over the net. Try to run your opponent, and he or she will do the same to you. It's a great drill for touch, angles, drop shots, and conditioning, because you are running a lot. Play points using this drill.
4. Play using only the service courts. Any ball hit deeper than the service line is out. Hit the ball easy and within the singles lines. Use either one or two service courts.

9 *Net Play*

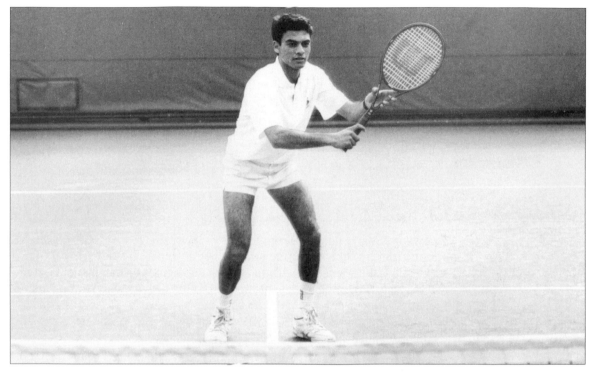

Outline

Many aggressive tennis players want to play the game at the net. Once you get to the net, you greatly increase the number of angles to which you can hit. And while the ball may come back quickly, the net player has great opportunities to put those balls away.

The Volley

A volley is the shot you make when you are near the net. In a volley, the ball does not touch the ground before you hit it. It is different from any other stroke. Four major differences follow:

1. The racket must be held farther in front of you, with your hands chest high and the racket head even with your eyes.
2. You should be facing the net with your head out in front of your shoulders and your shoulders in front of your feet. Eyes should be on a level with the ball, watching it intently from the moment it leaves your opponent's racket.
3. Your knees should be flexed, your feet shoulder-width apart, and body weight balanced on the balls of your feet.
4. Your feet should keep shifting, stepping, shuffling, and moving constantly so you can get a jump on the ball.

Your best all-around positioning for the volley seems to be inside the service court, two-thirds of the way back from the net. If you are a slower player, move back closer to the service line. If you are fast and agile, you can move up to a point as close as one-third of the distance from the net. Tall players can position themselves closer to the net than shorter players. Also, pick a position based on your opponent's game. If you are playing someone who is able to lob the ball high effectively, play back further from the net.

The ready position

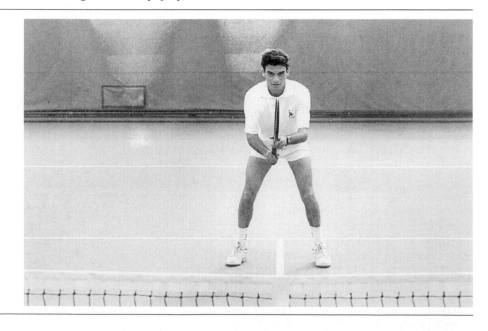

Forehand Volley

The grip for your forehand volley can be the regular eastern forehand or the continental. The eastern is best for beginners and intermediates, because you don't have the time to change grips. Higher-level players should use the continental, because it offers more control, feel, and backspin on the ball. Because it is halfway between the forehand and backhand grips, the continental also allows you to move your hand either way very rapidly. Even though this shot is short and fast, you need the 1-2-3-4 count to make it work.

Four-Count System for Forehand Volley

Count One: The Backswing

The instant that the ball leaves your opponent's racket, *move your hands up and forward* so that your right hand is even with your head and your racket head is higher than that. For a forehand volley, move the racket out in front of you at a 45-degree angle. Move your left hand up when the right one goes up, and point it at the oncoming ball. Keep your hands parallel, palms facing each other and quite close together. Your hands and your head should form a triangle in front of your face. Remember that *the backswing is very short*—about a foot, because the hand moves upward only a few inches and the racket moves back just a few degrees.

**Count One:
The backswing**

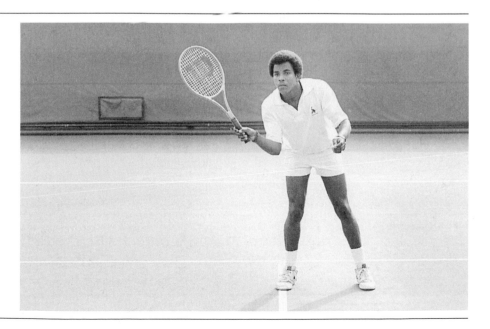

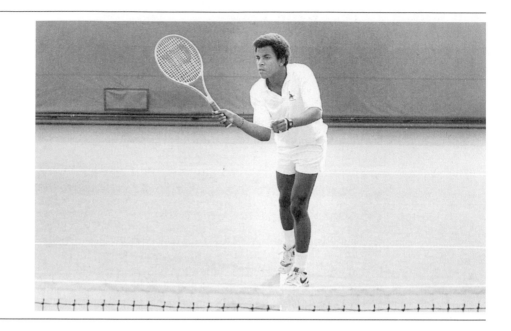

Count Two: The Step

Just after you raise your racket, *step forward to meet the ball.* If your feet have been moving, and you have time, step toward the net on your right leg, and then cross over to your left. If you are rushed, skip the right-leg step, and move to your left foot immediately. Always move forward toward the ball, shifting your weight to your left foot.

Other times, if you are fast enough, you can step out on the right foot, then cross over it with your left. Sometimes, however, the ball will be hit so hard you will only have time for the left step. Be careful not to let the racket move back behind your head as you move forward. Hold that tight triangle with head and hands close together and your head down on a steady line, leaning out over your body. It is important that you go after the ball rather than letting it come to you. It will give you a psychological lift and will also keep the ball from dropping low. Try to hit the ball when it is still high or rising.

Always keep your feet moving when you are in position to volley. You never know which direction you will have to move, back for an overhead or sideways or forward for a volley.

Count Three: Making Contact with the Ball

With your racket head above the ball and the racket hand about even with it, *punch down and out.* Don't stroke, swing, or even move your hand much more than a foot. Just move it forward to bring the racket down on the ball. Your arm and shoulder do very little work; the action stems mostly from your forearm.

Count Three: Making contact with the ball

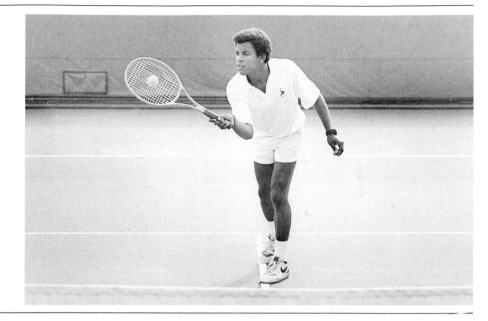

From backswing to ball contact, your hand shouldn't move more than a foot. To make sure you get backspin on the ball, hit it with the top edge of the racket slanted back a bit from the bottom edge. *Keep your head down and your eyes on the ball.*

Count Four: The Follow-Through

The racket head should be above your wrist when you hit the ball and about even when you've completed the short follow-through (about a foot). Keep your hand relaxed so you can feel the ball spin. Then lock your hand so the racket won't twist. At that point, your arm should be absolutely straight, but your wrist should be laid back a little. The racket head should be slanted just back a bit, strings toward the sky. The right amount of backspin will cause the ball to fade off and die when it contacts the ground. Make sure *you keep your racket through the ball* for 6 inches to a foot. Don't quit too soon.

The step forward and your natural momentum will carry you close to the net as you finish your follow-through. Get back to your original position fast so your opponent can't find you in a vulnerable position for a lob.

For the volley, get your hands up and your racket moving on Count One. Then, Count Two, Three, and Four are ticked off in a fast, continuous motion. The timing should be: 1—2-3-4. If you pause anywhere in the last three counts, your volley will not work.

Count Four:
The follow-through

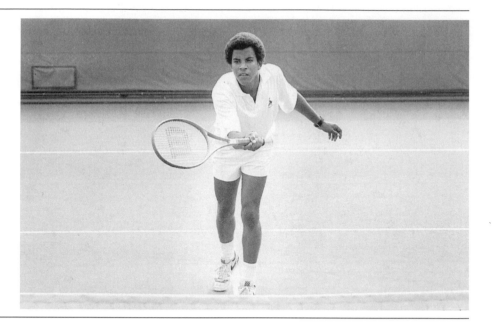

Forehand Volley Strategy

Picking up the low forehand volley is a science in itself. You need more back-spin to get that ball to pop up off your racket, clear the net, and come down deep in the other court. To do this, you have to bend your knees, get your eyes down level to the ball, and keep them there through the entire stroke.

Return of these low volleys is done with more racket touch and less power. Try to place the ball deep so it can't be put away while you are recovering to get into position. Putting it deeply into your opponent's backhand side is best.

On high volleys, remember to punch the ball; you don't need as much back-spin as on low volleys, because the ball is above the net. Every volley needs some backspin, unless you're an accomplished player who has mastered the flat volley.

If you are not sure whether the ball is going out or not, hit it; don't hesitate. If you have the time, go cross-court with your volley, because the backspin will make the ball skid when it hits the ground. But if you are in trouble and rushed, go to the deep backhand side, and make your opponent scramble for it.

When you are moving into the net after your serve and approach shot, put your first volley back deep, behind the service line. It's tough to make this first volley a winner, because you're running. You have a much better chance of making a point if you put this first volley deep at your opponent's weakest ground stroke (or backhand if his or her ground strokes are equal).

For those times when your opponent is way out of court, go to the open area. Otherwise, use your first volley so you can get into the net and put away the second or third volley. Watch the pros. They know that trying to put away every volley can lead to bad mistakes.

The full sequence for the forehand volley—right-handed player

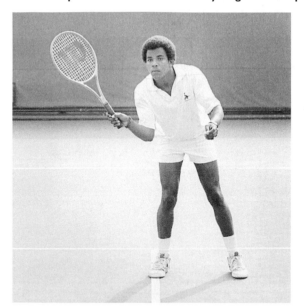

Count One: The backswing

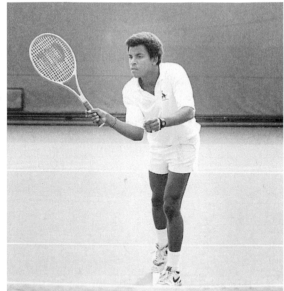

Count Two: The step

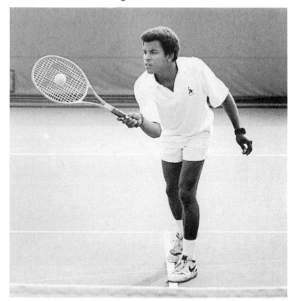

Count Three: Making contact with the ball

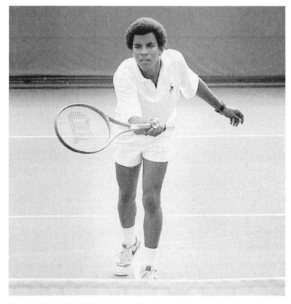

Count Four: The follow-through

The full sequence for the forehand volley—left-handed player

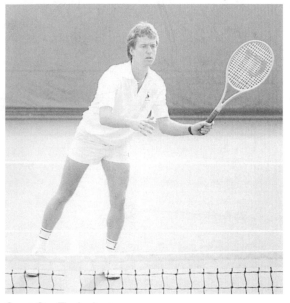

Count One: The backswing

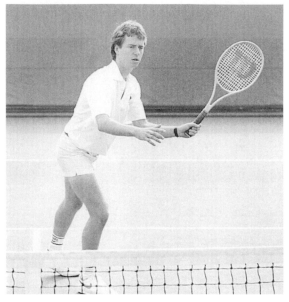

Count Two: The step

Count Three: Making contact with the ball

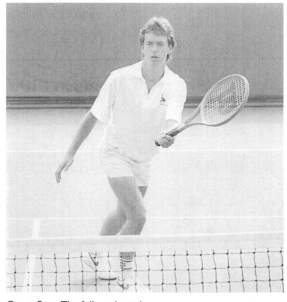

Count Four: The follow-through

Backhand Volley

The backhand volley ready position is much like that of the forehand. Remember to face the net, head out over your shoulders, shoulders leaning out over your feet. Stay up on the balls of your feet, and keep them moving. If you are a right-hander, cradle the racket with your left hand, keeping the left fingertips a few inches above your right hand.

When you see the ball coming to your backhand volley, change from your eastern forehand or continental grip to an eastern backhand or continental by lifting the right hand with the knuckle of the little finger toward you, letting your left hand twist the racket, and then grasping it again with the right hand. The left hand stays on the handle. A lot of players like the compromise continental grip for volleying.

Four-Count System for Backhand Volley

Count One: The Backswing

Keep your eyes on the ball, because you can't do anything until you see which direction the ball is going. Your feet and hands are signaled by your eyes, so watch the ball.

Most of the backswing for the backhand volley is identical to that of the forehand volley, except that you're going to the other side. As with the forehand, face the net and keep your feet moving. Move your hands up in front of your face, even with the oncoming ball as soon as it leaves your opponent's racket, as you did with your forehand. The racket head should be above your

**Count One:
The backswing**

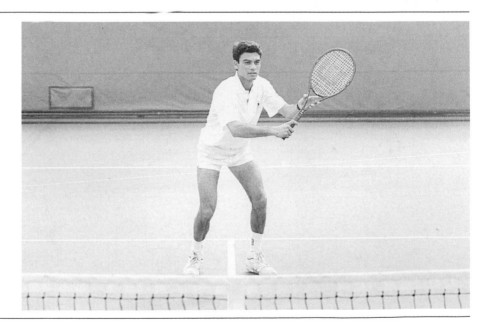

head about 45 degrees to the left and a little behind your hand. At no time in the volley backhand do your hands or arms go behind your body. Instead, they stay out in front of your face.

Count Two: The Step

Just before hitting the ball, shift your weight to your right leg, step toward the oncoming ball and the net, and turn your body a little sideways. Move forward toward the net, not sideways. If there's time, step out first with your left leg, and then cross over it with your right. If you're hurried, just step forward with the right leg.

Perfect timing would allow you to move your feet in little quick steps toward the ball, step out with the left leg, and then cross over with the right. Unfortunately, the speed of today's game seldom gives you the leisure for all of that, but whenever you can go through that entire series, do it. The result is much better position, balance, control, and approach to the ball.

When you turn slightly sideways, there will be a tendency to move your arms and hands behind your body. Fight that urge. Keep them out in front of your body. As with the forehand, don't wait for the ball to come to you, but go get it before it peaks over the net. The longer you wait, the less chance you have to hit the ball at its highest point. Catch the ball high, and step into it positively, up on your toes and stepping across with your right foot. Remember to get your eyes level with the ball and keep them there.

**Count Two:
The step**

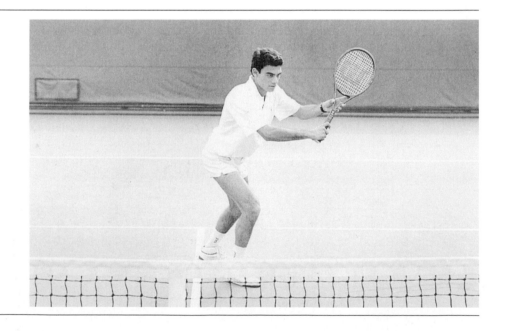

Count Three: Making contact with the ball

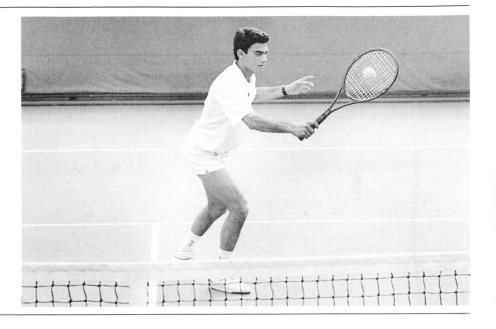

Count Three: Making Contact with the Ball

When you start forward with the racket head to make contact with the ball, release your left hand and straighten your right arm a little, turning your racket hand so the back of it faces away from you, toward the net. Bring the racket head out and down on the ball with the bottom edge leading.

At the moment of contact, the racket head should still be above the wrists. Your body should be leaning out over your right leg, with all of your weight on it. The left leg carries no weight at all. Move your head toward the ball, and keep your eyes on it all the way through the hit.

Count Four: The Follow-Through

For the entire backhand volley, your racket head moves only a couple of feet; and the follow-through takes up to a foot of that, but no more! At the completion of your follow-through, the racket head should be even with your wrist, and the bottom edge of the racket should be leading the top edge. For low volleys, the bottom edge will lead a little more, because you need more backspin to salvage the shot.

Your arm should be completely straight by now, but the racket ends up laid back a little at an angle from your arm. Make sure you get the backspin feel and go through the ball before recovering to get back into position. Don't ruin a good backhand volley by trying to recover too soon or by lifting your head and pulling up before you've finished the follow-through.

**Count four:
The follow-through**

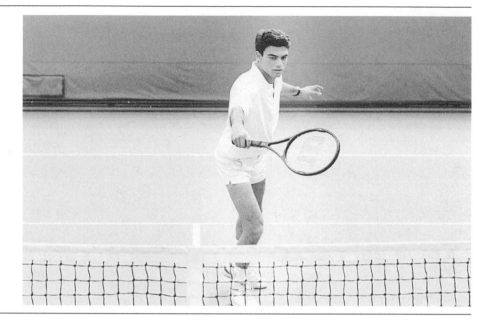

The backhand volley has the same 1 (pause)-2-3-4 rhythm as the forehand volley. It's backswing—then step, hit, follow-through. The last three counts come together in one fast routine.

Backhand Volley Strategy

There is a psychological reason for hitting a volley the way described here. Attacking the ball gives a player a positive response, while waiting for it seems to create a negative reaction—almost a fear of the ball. The key to a successful volley seems to be interception rather than reaction. "Get that ball before it gets you" is the motto.

When intercepting, try to hit the ball a bit harder than it was hit to you. This seems to reinforce that positive feeling. Don't, however, try to kill it to make every volley a put-away winner. This leads to expensive misses and mistakes. Low volleys are difficult to hit hard. But hit into those high ones for a feeling of self-confidence and game control.

Finally, practice your volley strokes as much as you do the ground strokes. A good volley can give you a balanced back-and-up (baseline and net) game and is worth practice equal time.

Forehand or backhand, don't try to put away that first volley when you are running into the net. It's too difficult a shot. Just keep the ball in play and deep; then, when you get to the net, punch hard or try placement of the volley for points. That opportunity might come on the second volley or the third or even the tenth, but don't try for the "sure" point until you are in a position to control your shot.

The full sequence for the backhand volley—right-handed player

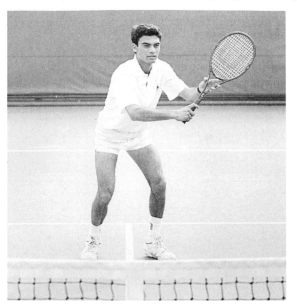

Count One: The backswing

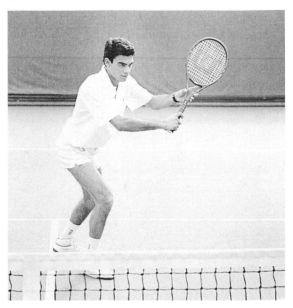

Count Two: The step

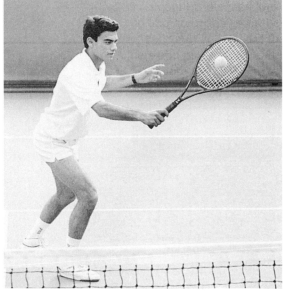

Count Three: Making contact with the ball

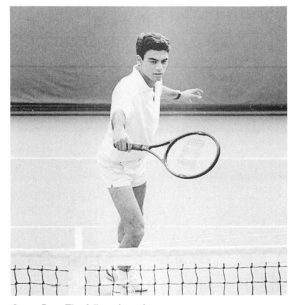

Count Four: The follow-through

The full sequence for the backhand volley—left-handed player

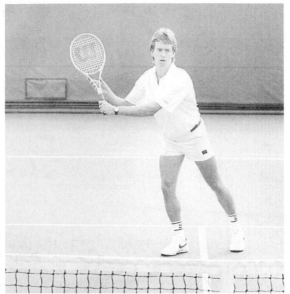

Count One: The backswing

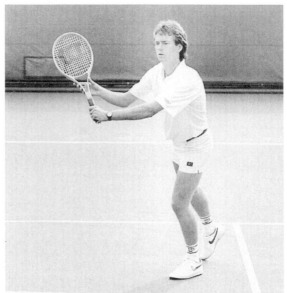

Count Two: The step

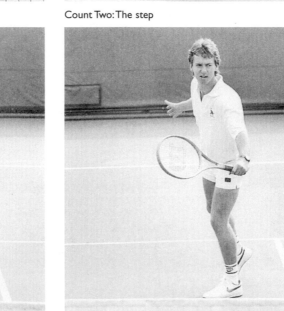

Count Three: Making contact with the ball

Count Four: The follow-through

> ✓ *Checklist for Forehand Volley—Right-Handed*
>
> 1. Get your racket up and into a good running position fast. Use a short back-swing, and get down low to the ball.
> 2. Move forward to intercept the ball before it comes to you. Go get the ball before it peaks over.
> 3. Just before contact, step across with your left leg and transfer your weight onto that leg.
> 4. With a short punching action, make contact with the ball. Use a slight under-spin hit.
> 5. Have a strong follow-through, then recover.
> 6. You need an aggressive attitude to be a good volleyer.

> ✓ *Checklist for Forehand Volley—Left-Handed*
>
> 1. Get your racket up and into a good running position fast. Use a short back-swing, and get down low to the ball.
> 2. Move forward to intercept the ball before it comes to you. Go get the ball before it peaks over.
> 3. Just before contact, step across with your right leg and transfer your weight onto that leg.
> 4. With a short punching action, make contact with the ball. Use a slight under-spin hit.
> 5. Have a strong follow-through, then recover.
> 6. You need an aggressive attitude to be a good volleyer.

Forehand and Backhand Half-Volley

A *half-volley* is a shot that is hit just after it bounces. Most tennis players agree that this is the toughest shot in tennis. Your timing must be perfect. Although the half-volley is played low (picked up within a foot of the ground), it is not played totally like a low volley.

To hit a successful half-volley, you must hit the ball just after it has hit the ground. Generally, you are up at the net, and your opponent slams one very fast right at your feet. You have a split second to get to it, under it, and lift it high enough to clear the net so it comes back down in the court yet is placed so it's not a put-away for your opponent.

Four-Count System for Half-Volley

Count One: The Backswing

Make sure you play the ball when it is in front of you. There is no wind-up on the backswing. Instead, you take the racket straight back a short distance, roughly half the distance of a ground stroke backswing. On the forehand, try to make a triangle with your hands and head. On the backhand, hold on to the racket with both hands. Don't raise the racket head above your wrist; instead, drop it below the wrist as it goes back. *Bend your knees*, and get down very low with body weight forward and balanced. *Keep your head down* to get a good look at the ball. If you must move to the ball, use small, quick steps so you don't overrun it or get yourself off balance.

Count Two: The Step

On the forehand side, try to step onto your left leg before hitting the ball. If you are running, you may not be able to do this, so hit off the right leg instead. On the backhand side, if you have time, step forward onto your right leg.

Count Three: Making Contact with the Ball

Get your racket head down under the ball, then lift the ball with a short, stroking action, putting enough topspin on the ball to get it over the net and back down into the court. Do not put backspin on this shot. Make sure your head and body stay down through the hit. If you look up, you are going to lift up and destroy the shot.

Count Four: The Follow-Through

Keep your racket on the ball for 6 inches to a foot after you contact it. End with a short follow-through, which goes only far enough to point where you're hitting. When finished, your racket should be higher than the contact point, and the top edge should be tilted forward slightly to help you put topspin on the ball. Make sure you have a strong follow-through. A blocking-only action won't work.

The full sequence for the half-volley—forehand

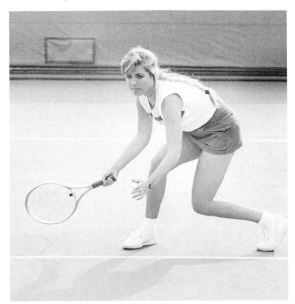

Count One: The backswing

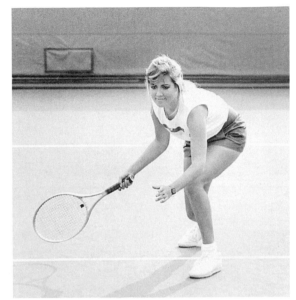

Count Two: The step

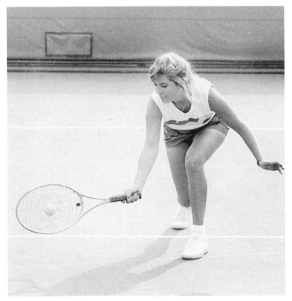

Count Three: Making contact with the ball

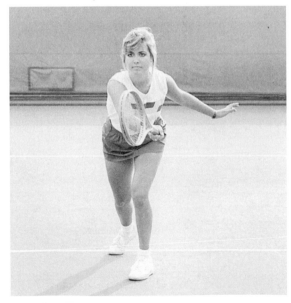

Count Four: The follow-through

The full sequence for the half-volley—backhand

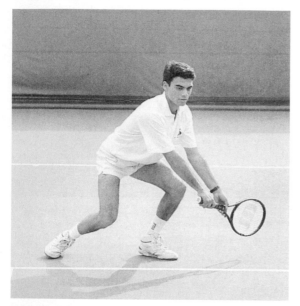

Count One: The backswing

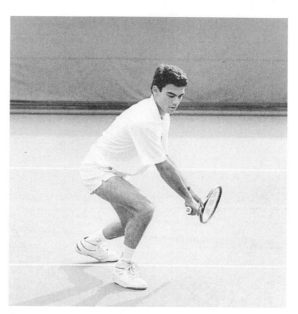

Count Two: The step

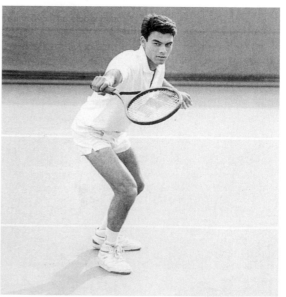

Count Three: Making contact with the ball

Count Four: The follow-through

Overhead Smash

The *overhead smash* is used when your opponent lobs the ball over your head to force you back deep into your court. If the lob is short, you have a great opportunity to attack your opponent with the smash.

The ready position is exactly the same as the volley ready position, and the grip is your choice of eastern forehand or continental. Most people prefer the eastern forehand for forehand overhead shots.

Four-Count System for Overhead Smash

Count One: The Backswing

When you see that lob coming, turn sideways, and get your feet moving toward the ball. Don't wind up as though you're going to serve, but instead, *run with both hands in the air* about head high. Your left hand should be aimed at the ball, and your right hand should be holding the racket up and ready for the hit. Turn your side toward the net, arms up, and move to the ball quickly.

Count Two: The Step

After using quick steps to *get behind the ball*, set up with the ball to the right and in front of you. Plant your right foot and push off, and step forward with your left foot. Keep your head up and eyes on the ball as you step forward. Keep your left arm pointing at the ball. Be careful not to pull your head or left arm down too soon, because you don't want to quit on this shot before it's completed.

Count Three: Making Contact with the Ball

The hitting action starts the way it does in the serve—by moving your right elbow up and forward. This cocks your wrist and also puts the racket down behind your back to provide the whip action you need for this shot. As with so many other strokes, don't wait for the ball to come to you. In this case, stretch to meet it. Keeping your head up and eye on the ball, swing the racket head flat through the ball. Occasionally, you can slice it cross-court, but most of the time you should hit this shot flat.

Count Four: The Follow-Through

Stay with the ball after you hit it, and control the direction of the ball by snapping your wrist and the racket head in the same direction. Finish the follow-through with the racket head coming down and across your left leg. The follow-through is just like your serve. Your racket follows through to your left side, and your right leg comes through naturally as you step forward on it.

The full sequence for the overhead smash

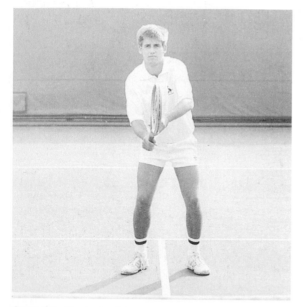

Count One: The backswing

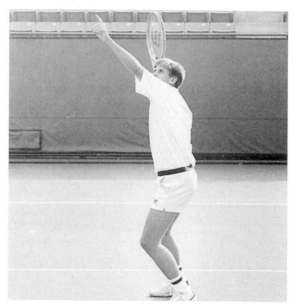

Count Two: The step

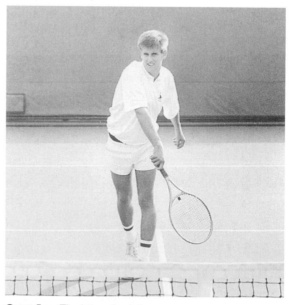

Count Three: Making contact with the ball

Count Four: The follow-through

✓ Checklist for Overhead Smash—Right-Handed Players

1. Move your feet before contact to keep the ball in front of you.
2. Use a short backswing.
3. Go up after the ball. Don't let it come down to you.
4. Your right shoulder should go up for contact and then forward after the contact.
5. Keep your left hand up, pointing at the ball, and be sure you see contact.

✓ Checklist for Overhead Smash—Left-Handed Players

1. Move your feet before contact to keep the ball in front of you.
2. Use a short backswing.
3. Go up after the ball. Don't let it come down to you.
4. Your left shoulder should go up for contact and then forward after the contact.
5. Keep your right hand up, pointing at the ball, and be sure you see contact.

Overhead Smash Strategy

Since your smash will be hit deep and hard, it is likely to keep your opponent off balance no matter where you hit it, but a shot at your opponent's feet or to the backhand side is most likely to win you the point.

Summary

1. The volley is a shot that is hit before the ball bounces. It is the most common shot used in net play.
2. To execute the volley:
   - Face the net, and keep your feet moving and your racket in front of you.
   - Keep your eyes on the ball.
   - Take a short backswing (about a foot).
   - Punch down and out at the ball with underspin.
3. The half-volley is a shot that is executed just after the ball has bounced.

4. To execute the half volley:
   - Keep your knees bent as you get down to the ball.
   - Keep your eyes on the ball.
   - Take a short backswing.
   - Put some topspin on the ball.
   - Take a short follow-through.
5. The overhead smash is used to attack when a player has lobbed the ball over your head.
6. To execute the overhead smash:
   - Run back to the ball with both hands up in the air.
   - As you get set to make your hit, point at the ball with your non-hitting hand (left hand for right-handers).
   - Hit the ball as you would a flat serve.
   - You don't have to put away all overheads—only the ones you are sure of. Be steady on the rest. Don't miss.

Drills for Players at All Levels

These drills are discussed further and illustrated in Chapter 14.

1. *Touch or Drop Volley.* With both players at the net, one feeds or hits to the other a low volley, which is then hit with an accentuated slicing action so that it stops or bounces back toward the net after it hits the ground. The drop-volleying player should almost catch the ball on the racket as the racket is cut sharply under the ball. You will need maximum spin and minimum speed on the ball as it barely clears the net. The advanced player will fake a hard shot before making the drop shot.

2. *Volleying* is best started with one player tossing or hitting to the forehand, then to the backhand of the volleyer. Later both players can volley gently— just hitting the ball, not trying to pass the opponent. Practice watching the ball. As you progress, start aiming for the corners of the service court—to increase the angle that your opponent must cover.

3. *Volleying Against the Wall* is a way to practice the volley without any help. Stand about 10 feet from the wall. First hit all forehand volleys, then all backhands, then alternate.

Drills for Intermediate and Advanced Players

These drills are discussed further and illustrated in Chapter 14.

1. *One Up–One Back.* This drill can be done forehand to forehand, backhand to backhand, or with a combination of shots. It can also be done with the net player hitting directly to the baseline player, but the baseline player hitting shots from side to side for the volleyer.

2. *Backcourt-Volley Combination* is started as a backcourt rally. When your opponent hits a short shot, attack the ball, make an approach shot, then volley.

3. *Reflex Volley Drill* has both players at the net. Keep the ball in the air; don't let it bounce. Both players should start at the service line and move in one step after each hit. Hit each shot at your opponent or at your opponent's feet—don't try for a sideline shot. Hit the ball with some backspin by hitting down on the ball with the racket face open.

4. *Overheads* are best started with one player tossing to the other, forcing the net player to run back, get in position behind the ball, then smashing it. The player hitting the overhead must return to the net after each smash, then move back to hit the next lob.

10 *Playing Against the Net-Player*

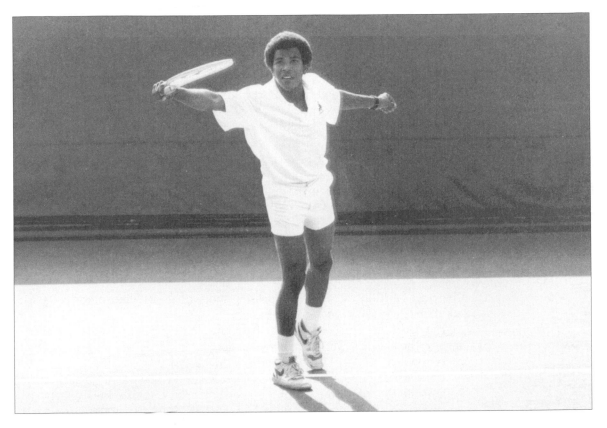

Outline

Passing Shots

The passing shot is a shot that passes your opponent when he or she is at the net. When you learn and master this stroke, you will be able to get the ball past the net-player in doubles and the net-rusher or volleyer in singles. If you don't learn it, your opponents are going to play the net and pick off your returns, slamming them for quick and easy points. It can be a tough shot to play properly, because you are usually on the run and don't have the time for perfect form.

Unlike the forehand and the backhand basic strokes, the passing shot is not intended as an ordinary return, but as a strategic shot calculated to win a point or at least put your opponent in a poor position to return the ball. Learn the following differences between this shot and the forehand and backhand basic strokes, plus the variations on the basic 1-2-3-4 count, and you are well on your way to "passing" with flying colors.

First, you should hit the ball harder and earlier than regular ground strokes. This robs your opponent of some of the time needed to get to your return. To hit the ball earlier, move up closer to the baseline when your opponent begins volleying. This moves you closer to the ball and lets you contact earlier. Also, hit the passing shot closer to the net than other shots.

Types of Passing Shots

There are basically three types of passing shots: down-the-line, hard-hit cross-court, and low, short cross-court.

The *down-the-line shot* should be hit with some topspin and a great deal of power. The idea is to get the shot by the net player before he or she can get a racket on it.

The second type, the *hard-hit cross-court*, is used when the net-player or volleyer starts getting your down-the-line shots. You can also use it effectively when the cross-court is open and unprotected. Hit with a little more topspin than the down-the-line.

The third passing shot, the *low, short cross-court*, is hit with a great deal of topspin if you are using your forehand. It is hit with the slice if you are using your backhand. Ideally, this return goes back crisply, but short and low, forcing the net-player to reach for the ball and make a bad volley that you can easily put away. Hit your backhand with topspin if you hit it two-handed.

Two-thirds of your passing shots should be those hard down-the-line blasts. Even if the shot doesn't get completely by the net-player, your opponent has less chance of putting it away for a point. Also, hitting a down-the-line shot on the run is easier than hitting cross-court.

To make your passing shot work properly, you need more topspin than you might use on other shots. This increased topspin will cause the ball to dip and drop suddenly as it crosses the net. If the ball is dropping, your opponent will have to hit it upwards to you, giving you an easy put-away.

Remember that the net is higher near the sidelines than in the center. Learn to compensate for this difference when hitting the down-the-line shots.

There is one more type of passing shot that is favored by advanced and tournament players: the *cannonball* is hit very hard and very directly at the net-player. Properly hit, this hard return should be aimed at the right hip of your right-handed opponents and the left hip of southpaws. By placing the ball at this location, you actually "handcuff" that opponent and prevent a forehand or backhand volley return. There is no practical way the racket can be positioned to pick a ball off the front of the hip.

Because you are usually running to make a passing shot, footwork is as important as racket work. The passing shot must be a better shot than other ground strokes, and you need position and balance to make it succeed. If you have time, or if you don't have to run very far to hit the passing shot, then your footwork should be the same as for the forehand or backhand ground stroke. When you are running, get there as fast as you can by taking longer strides and staying low so you won't have to take time to reposition your body for the stroke.

When running hard on the forehand side, hit in an open position (weight on your rear foot). This helps you get back into the court faster. Players on clay courts especially like the open position, since they can slide into the ball easier. The backhand return of the passing shot doesn't pose the same problem since your coiled body has a more naturally balanced position, even while running.

Four-Count System for Passing Shot

Count One: The Backswing

Because you are going to try hitting the ball harder and at an earlier position off the ground, take your racket back farther than the position you use for other ground strokes. Make sure you get that racket backswing started as soon as you see the ball leave the opponent's racket and as soon as you know whether you are going to need a forehand or backhand. On the forehand, remember to keep your left hand pointing out and your head low, eyes level with the oncoming ball.

Count Two: The Step

As you run down the ball, try to step into it with your front leg if possible. As you step forward to meet the ball, make sure your racket is back far enough to hit the ball hard, but not so far back that you are out of control. Remember, when on the run, hit the forehand off the right leg.

Count Three: Making Contact with the Ball

After you step, start uncoiling the racket by throwing the head out and toward the ball. Because you are going to hit the ball closer to the net, you don't have

The full sequence for the forehand passing shot—right-handed player

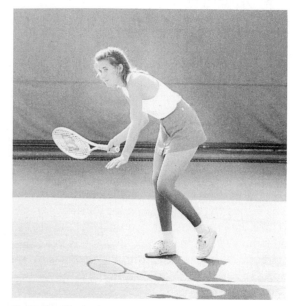

Count One: The backswing

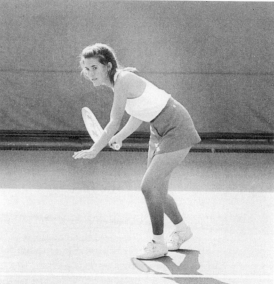

Count Two: The step

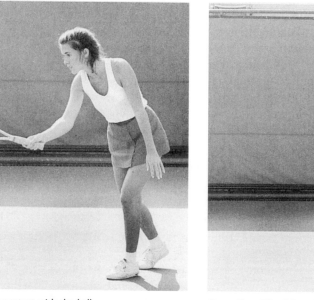

Count Three: Making contact with the ball

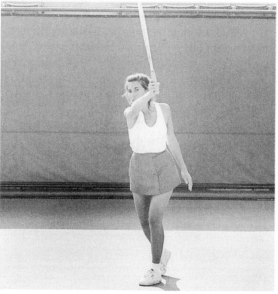

Count Four: The follow-through

to hit *up* on the ball so much in order to hit it over the net. Make sure you move out rapidly to attack the ball instead of letting it come to you. When you aggressively attack the ball, you develop a positive feeling of control. Waiting for the ball builds a negative feeling.

The full sequence for the forehand passing shot—left-handed player

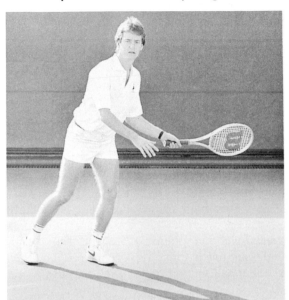

Count One: The backswing

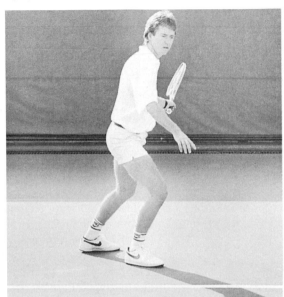

Count Two: The step

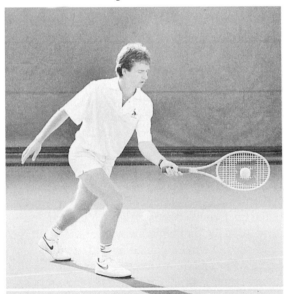

Count Three: Making contact with the ball

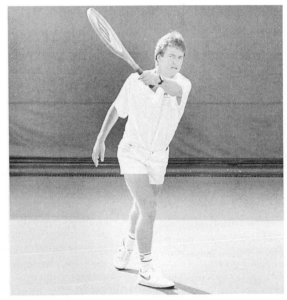

Count Four: The follow-through

Count Four: The Follow-Through

Maintain contact with the ball for 6 inches to a foot when you start your follow-through. During this period, your racket head moves in the direction you want the ball to go. After the ball leaves the racket head, your arm should be straight. It moves past the intended line of flight as your shoulder comes forward to touch your chin. If you used topspin, then the arm should end up a little bent, and the racket will be higher than usual.

Lobs

The *lob* can be one of the secret weapons of winning tennis. But many players, even advanced ones, mistakenly believe that it is a last-ditch, or desperation, shot for the amateur. You can throw your opponents completely off by lobbing a great deal at the start of the match. High, deep lobs, cleverly mixed with your other ground strokes, should keep your opponents scurrying back from the net and finally confuse their net-volleying game.

There are two basic types of lobs: the defensive and offensive. They require somewhat different techniques. Learn them both and practice them as regularly as your other strokes.

Don't let the terminology of "defensive" and "offensive" fool you. The offensive lob can be hit when you are desperately trying to retrieve the ball, and the defensive lob can be used when you are all set and could have easily used another type of ground stroke.

Four-Count System for Defensive Lob

Count One: The Backswing

The defensive lob is most often used to save a point you might otherwise lose. Suppose your opponent has hit a well-placed shot, and your only chance to recover is to keep the ball in the court and in play. To do that, you have to start moving extra fast when you see the ball leave your opponent's racket. Get your racket low, because the defensive lob needs to be hit both high and deep.

Count Two: The Step

When you are running to the forehand side, it is almost impossible to hit your return off the front leg. Instead, step back onto your back leg. This helps you get low and under the ball and also keeps you moving away from the net to get more time for your return. An extra second can be gained by letting your body fall back over that back leg and give with the ball as you begin your swing.

On the backhand side, you should usually "give" with the ball off your back leg, but you should still fall back away from the net to give yourself more time to get under it.

Count Three: Making Contact with the Ball

When you step back, get that racket head totally under the ball before starting your hit. The racket head should come up flat, almost parallel to the ground. Hit

The full sequence for the forehand defensive lob

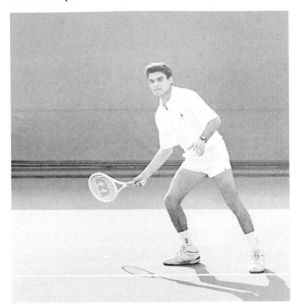

Count One: The backswing

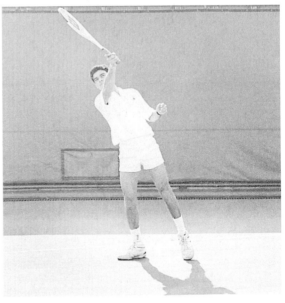

Count Two: The step

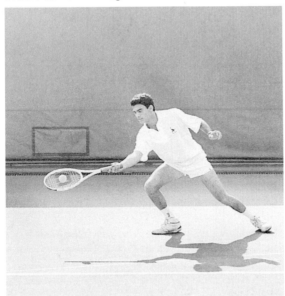

Count Three: Making contact with the ball

Count Four: The follow-through

the ball at any height you can get it, even scooping it that last inch before it can bounce twice. Straighten your body as you make contact with the ball. This gives you the power you need for arc and depth. If you are making a desperation reach, however, your arm will have to do the work.

The full sequence for the backhand defensive lob

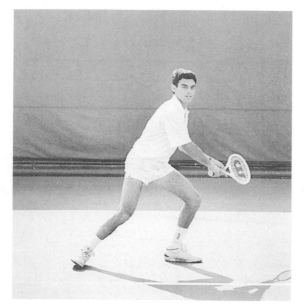

Count One: The backswing

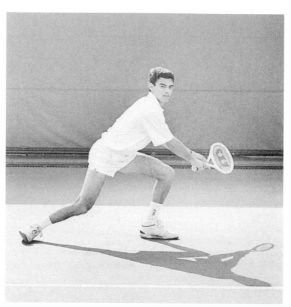

Count Two: The step

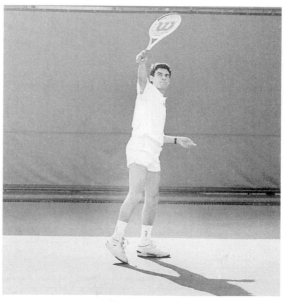

Count Three: Making contact with the ball

Count Four: The follow-through

The ball is usually hit flat. One exception is when you are reaching for the ball on the backhand side. Here the slice action might be more effective. Also, when the opponent has smashed an overhead directly at you, and you are cramped for swinging room and time, the slice might save the shot.

Count Four: The Follow-Through

Hit straight up, about perpendicular to the ground. Your racket should end up high; higher than any other shot. Continue straightening up while you fall back and away from the net. If you can jump off the ground, do it. This gives you extra power for arc and depth on this shot.

Finally, don't try to scramble back into the court until you have regained your balance. You have plenty of recovery time because your opponent can't get to the ball until it comes down, and a good high lob can take forever to come back down to the court.

Defensive Lob Strategy

The basic use of the defensive lob is to keep the ball in play and not give your opponent that point. It is a good defensive maneuver and is used by the pros and by advanced players to salvage a bad situation. Here are some tips on how you too can do that.

- Be sure to aim your lob for the middle of the opponent's court and deep. It is a mistake to try for accurate placement because you are usually scrambling for the shot, and your return can easily go out of bounds.

- Stay away from the defensive lob when the wind is at your back. Those breezes too often carry the ball outside the court. On the other hand, use it a great deal when the wind is against you. You can smite it a mighty blow and the wind should still keep it in the court.

- Use the sun. A high, arcing lob is hard for your opponent to follow when the sun is in his or her eyes. Don't overlook such aspects of the weather when they can add to your game.

- The higher and deeper you hit the ball, the more time your opponent might have to wait for it to bounce. While your opponent is waiting, you will have plenty of time to get back into the court and ready for your next shot. Also, remember that the deeper you hit it, the farther back from the net your opponent has to move to play it.

- Because the lob is a slow, time-consuming stroke, this change of pace can often unnerve your opponent, especially the quick, impatient type of player. Given time to think about a shot, many of these players will tense up and miss it.

- Use the lob to discourage your opponent. No player can stay enthusiastic if his or her returns are consistently chased down and lobbed back. A sort of psychological weariness will set in eventually, and your opponent will start missing.

- The lob is a good way to wear your opponent down physically. The overhead smash is a tiring, wearing shot and a series of high lobs requiring those overhead smashes will have the same effect on an opponent as body punches do on a boxer.

Four-Count System for Offensive Lob

The offensive lob differs from the defensive because it is much lower. The defensive lob is usually done to gain time. The offensive lob is used to gain a point by hitting over a close net-player.

Count One: The Backswing

If you are going for a forehand offensive lob, take your racket back exactly the way you do for a passing shot. For a backhand lob, take the racket back as though you are going to slice. Keep your backswing short, so you stay balanced as you run and can get to the ball without reaching.

Count Two: The Step

Count Two is the most important of the four counts because it's here that you can outfox your opponent. Act as though you are going to hit a passing shot, which is what is expected, instead of the lob. You can mislead your opponent by exaggerating your step, coiling your body as though for a passing shot. Keep your head down. If you lift too soon, you signal that you are going to lob. This type of faking should cause a good, experienced opponent to move forward to intercept that expected volley. One caution: Don't be such a good faker that you fake yourself out.

Count Three: Making Contact with the Ball

The idea of the offensive lob is to get the ball just over the reach of the net-player. It shouldn't be too high, because a higher ball gives your opponent time to retreat and retrieve.

Aim the shot higher than you would for a normal forehand or backhand. If you can use topspin, do it. You need to hit the ball more underneath than you would for a regular shot, and you need to finish higher.

Because you are hitting a lob, there is a tendency to raise your head to give the ball more topspin and more lift. Resist that tendency.

Count Four: The Follow-Through

Don't pull up too soon. Try to stay with the ball for a few inches to maintain better control and help deceive your opponent. Swing the racket so it finishes a little higher than the final position for a passing shot. On the forehand, the racket should end up more closed, because of the topspin. For the backhand, it should finish more open, because of the slice.

Don't hold this follow-through very long, because you have to get back into the court to prepare for two possibilities: One, if you didn't hit the shot very well, you've given your opponent an easy overhead return; two, even if you did hit it

The full sequence for the forehand offensive lob

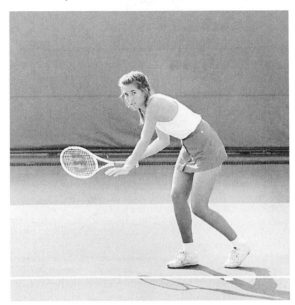

Count One: The backswing

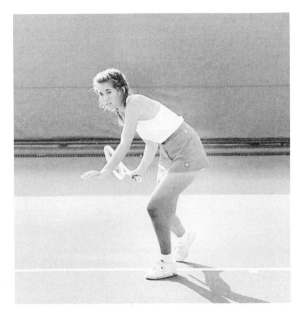

Count Two: The step

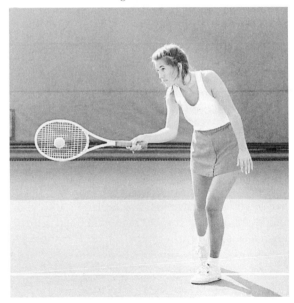

Count Three: Making contact with the ball

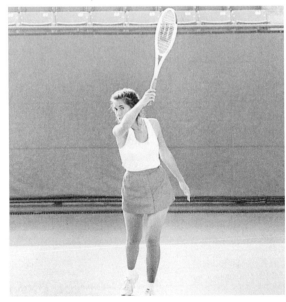

Count Four: The follow-through

> **✓**   *Checklist for the Lob*
>
> 1. Hit the lob high and deep.
> 2. Don't let your opponent know you are going to lob until the last minute (move as if you are going to make a passing shot).
> 3. Aim for the middle of the court if you are running hard to give yourself some tolerance.
> 4. Make your follow-through high.

well, he or she might still get to and return it. If the ball does get over your opponent's head, get up to the net fast and be ready for any type of return.

Offensive Lob Strategy

The offensive lob is a strong answer to someone who tries to control the net or easily picks off your passing shots. It can be effective at other times, too. For example, when your opponent has made a great shot from the back court and put you in trouble, a lob to that back court can give you more time to recover and reposition yourself.

There are three times to avoid using the offensive lob. If you have the time and position to hit a passing shot instead of the lob, do it. The percentages are greater that the passing shot will work. Also, never use the lob shot against a poor player. The lob is a lower percentage shot for you than is a passing shot. Finally, don't use it against a poor volleyer. Force that person to volley by hitting passing shots to him. Eventually the poor player will be poorer by one point.

Against a good player who volleys well, however, you should start throwing up lobs to drive your opponent back from the net. The farther back you can move your opponent, the tougher it is for him or her to get off a good volley return.

When you start gaining control of your offensive lob, begin placing it to your opponent's backhand. It is extremely hard to put away a high backhand return. You will usually get a soft, somewhat out-of-control return, which you should be able to put away for a point.

Strategy for Playing Against the Net-Player

1. When you are in the back court and your opponent is at the net, you are at a disadvantage. Passing shots and lobs, though lower-percentage shots, are ways that you can turn the tables.
2. Whenever you can make points from a disadvantageous position, you are in command of the match. For that reason, you should practice attacking the net-player.

The full sequence for the backhand offensive lob

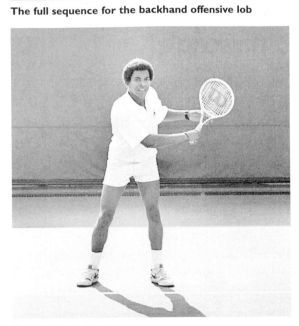

Count One: The backswing

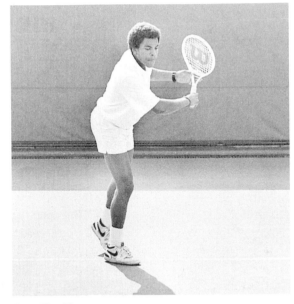

Count Two: The step

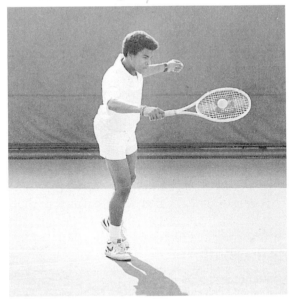

Count Three: Making contact with the ball

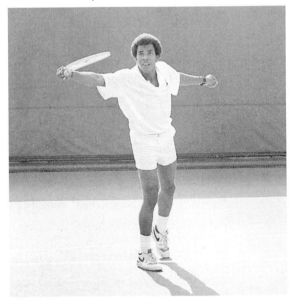

Count Four: The follow-through

3. Passing shots can be made down the line, deep cross-court, or shallow cross-court.

4. For the passing shot:
   - Take your racket straight back, a little further than for a regular ground stroke.
   - Bend at the knees to get down to the ball.
   - Shift your weight on your forward leg to assure full power.

5. Defensive lobs are generally used to save a point that you might otherwise lose and to give yourself time to get back into position. For defensive lobs:
   - Take a short backswing while keeping your racket very low.
   - "Fall away" from the shot as you hit it by allowing more weight to move to your back foot.
   - Hit straight up.
   - Aim to the deep middle of your opponent's court.

6. Defensive lobs should be used more often if the sun is high to your back (so that it will be in your opponent's eyes) or if you are hitting into the wind.

7. Offensive lobs should just clear your opponent's reach. They should be executed to look like a ground stroke.

Summary

1. There are three ways to pass an opponent who is at the net. The down-the-line shot should be used most often. Cross-court shots or short cross-court angle shots should be used about a third of the time.

2. A more advanced shot, the cannonball, is hit directly at the right hip of a right-handed opponent.

3. Lob shots are a way to get a net-player to move back from the net.

4. The defensive lob shot helps to buy you time. It is hit high over the net-player, forcing him or her to retreat past the baseline.

5. The offensive lob is a way to get a point by just clearing your opponent's racket but not giving him or her time to get back in position to play your shot.

Drills for Players at All Levels

These drills are discussed further and illustrated in Chapter 14.

1. *Lobs* can be practiced with one player hitting to the other. Start with defensive (high) lobs, then work with offensive (low) lobs.

2. *Lob-Overhead Combination* is done with one player lobbing and the other hitting overheads. The person hitting the overheads can come to the net and touch it with the racket after the hit. This forces a return to the net position while it increases physical conditioning.

11 *Singles Play Strategy*

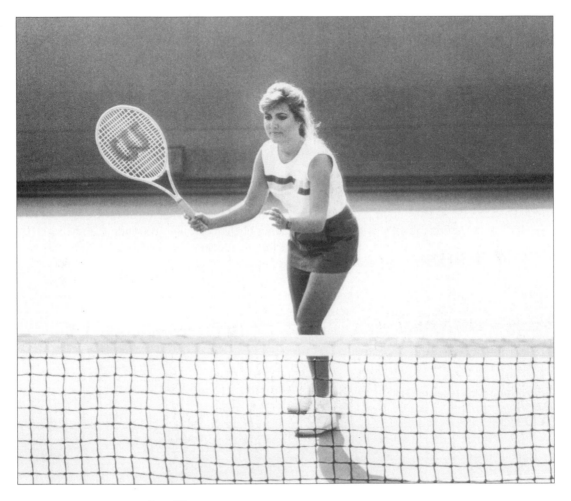

Outline

Y ou will improve your chances of winning at singles play if you do not attempt to do more than you know you are capable of at your present level of skill. "Showboating," or trying for great shots you know you can't make, only leads to disappointment, lost games, and a general erosion of self-confidence. Instead of trying to "kill" your opponent with one fantastic passing shot, stay with the shots you can handle. Let your opponent make the mistakes and give you the points.

Rallies

One of the major purposes of a rally is to move your opponent out of position. To stay in court and in command, keep the ball deep. It doesn't matter if you hit it 5 feet over the net as long as it lands near the baseline. Remember that the closer your shot is to the net, the greater the chance it will be returned. So play conservatively during a rally. Just get the ball in.

Back Court Rallies

Most back court rallies are backhand-to-backhand, because cross-court back-hands are easy and safe to hit. Generally, you should be standing anywhere from 2 to 10 feet behind the baseline; the deeper you are, the steadier you can be. If you want to develop more offense or hit deeper shots, move up, possibly inside the baseline if your opponent starts to have trouble. However, if you have hit a weak backhand cross-court, return behind the baseline to give your-self more time and room to run down the return.

Back court position for back court rally

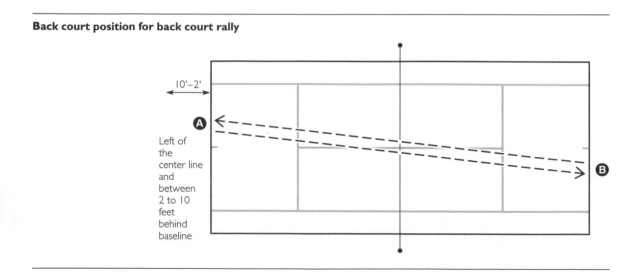

10'–2'

Left of
the
center line
and
between
2 to 10
feet
behind
baseline

Back court position for forehand rally

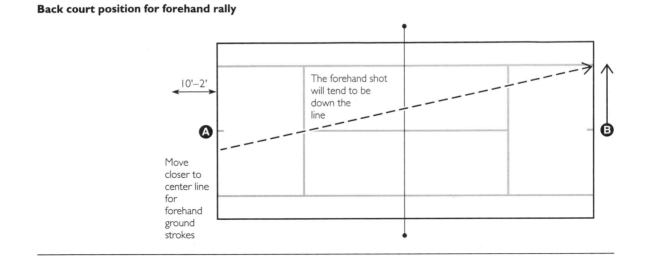

In addition to standing deep, start your backhand rally standing a little to the left of the center line. If your opponent is like most players, he or she will have a difficult time hitting backhands down the line to your forehand and will tend to go cross-court to your backhand instead. Standing to the left of the center gives you a better angle on the ball without totally surrendering the forehand court.

When you get off a good backhand shot that forces your opponent to scurry and stretch, then move over to the right of center and inside the baseline a little. That is probably where the weak return will end up, and you should be waiting for it.

If you hit a short, poor backhand cross-court, your opponent might very well come in and hit a down-the-line approach shot. Be prepared for this, and balance the court by moving to your right. Also, watch for the drop shot.

When you hit a forehand cross-court to your opponent's forehand, stand nearer to the center line. For backhands cross-court, move to the left a bit. Again, if your opponent is like most players, he or she will tend to hit forehands down the line more often than backhands down the line.

Regarding depth, if you are trying simply to play a steady rally to move your opponent around and make him or her tired, play those rallies from behind your baseline. But if you are hitting offensively and getting off hard shots, move up to within a foot or two of the baseline.

When you do achieve an excellent shot that forces your opponent to reach, move inside the baseline and a bit to the side of your shot to pick off the return. Remember, however, when you are forced into a weak return, hasten deep into the back court area because your opponent is probably going to smack a deep approach shot. But always be alert for the short drop shot.

Passing shots against the net-player

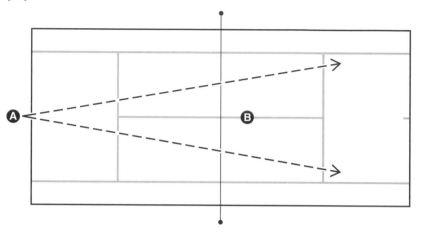

Playing Against the Net-Player

Don't be intimidated by your singles opponent coming to the net. Many players do this in the hope it will cause panic and, consequently, mistakes. Too often, they are right. Instead of watching your opponent, watch the ball and play your own shot. If you don't panic, and if you don't try to put the ball away each time you stroke it, you'll get a better than fair share of points.

When a very steady player comes up to the net against you, if you make that player volley again and again, you should eventually get the point. For some reason, most steady players don't volley very well. If you continue getting the ball back to them, they will eventually make a mistake.

On the other hand, if you are playing against a superb volleyer, then your only chance of victory is an effective group of passing shots.

Positioning at the Net

If you have the skills to play at the net, it is definitely better to do so. When you play at the baseline, you have about a 19-degree angle for your shots. At the net, the angle can increase to as much as 130 degrees. And since tennis is a game of angles, the wide angle is better than the narrow angle.

What are your strengths and weaknesses? If you are tall, you should probably play close to the net; likewise, if you volley and hit overheads well. If you have a powerful or tricky serve, you should also be able to follow it to the net.

If you hit good ground strokes, can lob effectively, and are in good physical condition, perhaps you should concentrate on the back court game. If you are a poor server, you won't be able to follow your serve in. You will have to play the

Angle increases as you approach net

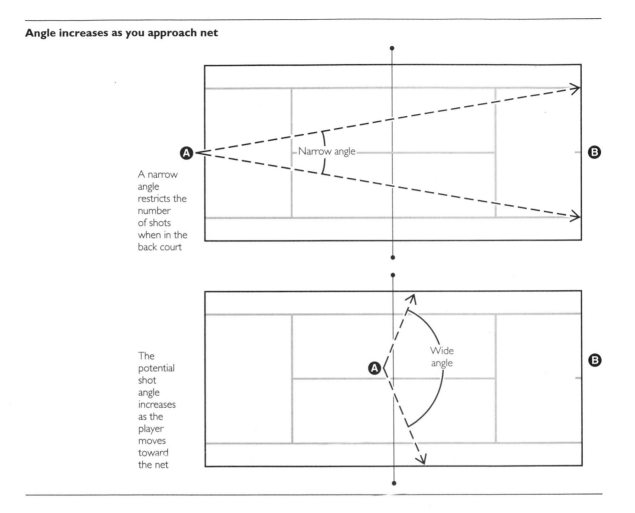

A narrow angle restricts the number of shots when in the back court

Narrow angle

The potential shot angle increases as the player moves toward the net

Wide angle

back court and wait until your opponent has hit a short, weak shot before you can take the net.

The way your opponent plays also determines where you should play. If your opponent has effective ground strokes, then it is to your advantage to move that player up to the net using angled shots or drop shots. If, on the other hand, your opponent has weak ground strokes, then keep him or her in the back court by hitting the ball deep to different sides. Then you can come up to the net yourself to put away those easy ground strokes that are being sent back. Obviously, if your opponent has a strong serve, you move back away from the baseline, while a weak serve demands that you move up, even into the court. So, you see, the way your opponent plays helps determine your position.

Furthermore, most tennis players have habits or tendencies that you can take advantage of by your position. For example, if your opponent is very fond of the forehand cross-court shot, position yourself to the right of center on your court, and you can start adding up your points. If, however, your opponent tends to go down the line with backhands, position yourself in that direction. Of course, if you overadjust on any of these moves, you could put yourself completely out of position for the next return. To adjust properly, move over just enough to give you the advantage but not far enough to pull you out of position. For the opponent who loves to throw up those skyball lobs, play back from the net.

The idea is to take away whatever your opponent does best and make him or her switch strategies and play weaker shots. Often you will have to get to an opponent's weak shot through a strong shot. For example, if your opponent has a weak backhand while running, hit a wide forehand; then your next shot goes to the backhand.

Try to read what your opponent is going to hit and where. Pros and advanced players can often anticipate the coming shot from the action of their opponent's racket. If the racket head drops while the player is stepping out to meet the ball, chances are the return will go cross-court. If you anticipate it, you can be there, smiling, ready for a slick return.

When the ball gets behind your opponent and he or she is trying to slice it, it will either go down the line or up into a lob. Learn to read the angle, speed, and attitude of the racket head in order to get a jump on the oncoming ball. However, don't depend on this type of "reading" totally. It is wiser to learn your particular opponent's individual habits. Watching your opponent warm up will give you some clues.

As a general rule, play in the center of your baseline when in the back court, and play between the ball and the center of your baseline whenever you move toward the net. This will keep your court "balanced." Try to keep your court balanced as much as possible, and take advantage of an unbalanced oppo-

Keep court balanced playing in back court

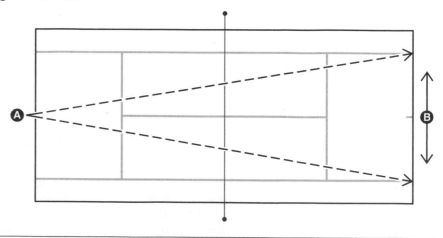

Keep court balanced playing at net

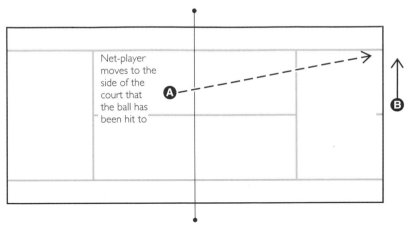

Net-player moves to the side of the court that the ball has been hit to

nent's court to score points. When you are balanced, you can play either side. When you are out of position, you open up a large part of your court for your opponent's shots.

Where your opponent moves after hitting a shot can be important to the way you should play it; therefore, advanced players not only watch the ball coming in, but also observe where the other player is moving. If your adversary is not coming into the net, you can reach the ball and make a nice, steady shot without hurrying. If your opponent is coming in to the net, your shot must be better planned and stroked to avoid its being returned.

One other advantage of taking a split second to observe the other player is to see if he or she is in trouble. A player out of position or out of control can be an easy target for a well-placed shot to the open side of the court.

Caught out of position, many players foolishly just give up and abandon the point to the other person. Instead, if you are caught out of position, try faking a move one way and then the other just before your opponent hits the ball. If his or her reflexes aren't fast enough, you may find the return shot just where you want it. A clever variation of this is to fake one way, start the other, then stop and stay where you are. Sometimes your opponent will become confused and hit the ball right back to you. However, this is a risky maneuver that could backfire, so try it only when you are in real trouble.

Playing at the Net

When you serve or make an approach shot and come to the net while your opponent is still in the back court, you need position adjustments to handle the returns. If you have hit to the forehand side, move to the left of the center line.

If your shot moves your opponent way out of court, move a yard or so to the left, because chances are the return will come down the line on that side. When you have hit the ball to the backhand side, move right a little, especially if your opponent is in trouble. The closer you play to the net, the easier it is for you to control the game. But watch out for the lobber. An opponent who can throw up successful lobs is an opponent who can hurt your net game.

Playing from the Back Court

In the reverse situation, where your opponent is at the net and you are in the back court, play close to the baseline. If a ball is hit to your backhand, move over to hit the ball, then swiftly return to your center position to balance the court. The same holds true when you hit a cross-court passing shot either with your backhand or forehand. Every time you are forced out of that center base-line position by your opponent's placement or your return, scuttle back there quickly to balance the court. If you manage a good passing shot that catches your opponent unprepared, move into the court to receive what will probably be a weak volley that you can hit away for a winner.

Positioning for Best Shots

- For safe, steady ground strokes, position yourself 2 to 10 feet behind the baseline. For harder hits or a stronger attack, move closer to the baseline or even inside it.
- To hit offensive volleys for put-aways, play close to the net. In this position, be alert for lobs.
- On the overhead shot, run to a position in which you can hit the ball while it's in front of and to the right of you. Try not to reach for it, but do keep moving forward when you hit. When returning a high overhead that comes down near your baseline, let it bounce first to give yourself a better return and better position for the next shot.
- If you are positioned at the baseline, don't hit the drop shot unless you're trying to bring your opponent up to the net. The best time to hit the drop shot is when you are at the service line or even closer to the net.
- Stay away from the approach shot when you're deep or behind the baseline. It takes too long for you to get to the net. The ideal place to stroke this shot is when you are close to the net—the closer the better. Wait until you get a short return before using your approach shot.
- On the serve, changing position occasionally at the baseline can confuse your opponent and upset his or her timing. Stand close to your center line and serve down the middle of your opponent's service courts to gain points. Moving out from that center line gives you stronger angles. Remember, an imaginary line drawn across your toes will show you the angle at which the

Position against strong versus weak server

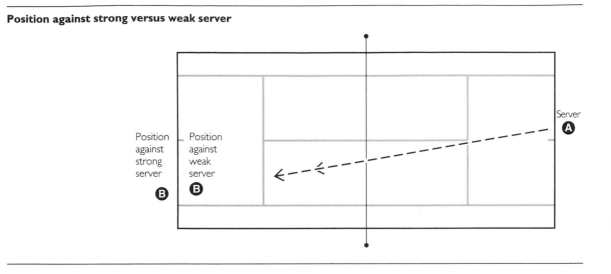

serve will go. If you miss the first serve, play the second one from the spot that's giving you the highest percentage of successful ones.

- Having trouble with your opponent's serve? Move back to give yourself more time and room to get it. If the serve is slow or uncertain, move in to attack it. Most players have service habits. If the server tends to serve wide, for example, play wide. If he or she hits a lot of center line shots, play there. If the serves are often to your backhand, adjust to be prepared for them. If you deliberately position yourself very deep or very wide to the right or left, your opponent will often have trouble with depth perception or perspective. If you can make the server focus on watching you, always wondering where you will be, you may cause your opponent to lose concentration on the serve and thus miss more often.

- Move up close to the baseline for passing shots so that you can hit the ball on the rise.

- Position yourself at or just inside the baseline to hit offensive lobs. This gets the ball over your opponent's head with no time to recover for an overhead smash. For defensive lobs, however, get far back behind the baseline so you can get under the ball, hit it hard, and still have time to recover back into court.

- If you hit a defensive lob and you're somewhat out of position, then throw up a high lob that will give you time to get back into court balance.

✓ *Checklist for Singles Play Strategy*

1. Always change your strategy if you are losing.
2. Keep the ball in play. Don't beat yourself.
3. Look for your opponent's weaknesses.
4. Know what you can and cannot do.
5. Go to the net more against a net rusher.
6. Bring the baseline player up to the net more often than he or she wants.
7. Play every point as if it were match point.
8. Attack more often on fast courts and play steady on slow courts.
9. Mix up your spins.
10. Keep the ball deep on back court rallies.
11. Lob whenever you are in trouble.

Footwork

The single most important rule is to keep your feet moving all the time. The only tennis player who should be standing around is somebody who is waiting for a court!

It may be a long distance between your head and feet, but nothing controls your footwork more than your eyes. Your feet can't see the ball coming, so your eyes have to tell them. This eye-foot communication is so important that some slower-moving players with good eyes can reach the ball much faster than faster players with lazy eyes. Total visual alertness is absolutely necessary to a good tennis player.

Good footwork opens up opportunity shots. For example, if you hit a backhand, then stand around watching its graceful flight, you won't be ready to return your opponent's weak shot. If you'd been moving, your answer to the weak return could easily be a passing shot or an advantageous approach shot. When you're moving, short balls are perfect for put-aways; but if you're not moving, they can plop in for points. Getting to the ball earlier and faster gives you the opportunities to make strong offensive shots out of weak defensive ones.

Getting a jump on the ball by using your eyes gives you a chance to glide instead of running hard to retrieve it. When you hit a ball on the run, your eyes aren't usually set and you don't get a good look at it. Gliding for the ball keeps your head and eyes from bobbing up and down, keeps your strokes steadier, and even conserves strength.

For ground strokes, there are three basic ways to move to the ball. With all of them, you move your body to face the net as much as possible and hold your racket in the beginning of the backswing position. Although you may have to partially turn to run after a ball, try keeping your body facing the net. Going to the forehand side, step out first with the outside leg (the right). For the backhand side, step out first with the left.

If a shot is at you, step back with the first step, then step into the ball with the second. So, for a right-handed forehand, step behind with the right foot back and to the left about 2 feet. Then step forward with the left foot. For a backhand, step behind with the left foot, then forward with the right.

Consistency in good strokes is one of the secrets of a good tennis player, and consistency in footwork is the secret behind that secret. Moving quickly and effectively helps you produce consistently good strokes. You can hit the same stroke the same way and therefore continually perfect it if your footwork is good. Bad footwork, however, will force you to hit behind you one time, out in front of you another, or handcuff you a third. You can't develop a good ground-stroke game if you can't hit the ball the correct way. Being there and being ready for the ball is the best way to develop ideal strokes.

Summary

1. Position yourself to take away your opponent's advantages—whether that position is right or left, front or back.
2. Make your opponents play with their weaker shots. Don't let your opponents play their game. You control the game instead.
3. Remember that the general rule is to play in the middle of your baseline, or between that spot and the ball if you are in front of the baseline. And the specific rule is to watch the ball and move *as*, not after, you see it.
4. Keep your feet moving.
5. Generally play conservatively.
6. When rallying, hit the ball deep, usually to the backhand.
7. When your opponents are at the net, play to their weaknesses and away from their strengths. Make the poor volleyer hit volleys. Make the good volleyer hit passing shots and lobs.
8. Position yourself to take advantage of the tendencies of your opponent. For example, play more to the backhand side if that is where your opponent likes to hit the ball.

Drills for Players at All Levels

These drills are discussed further and illustrated in Chapter 14.

1. *Down-the-Line Passing Shot.* The baseline player hits to the net-player, who hits to a deep corner. The baseline player attempts to hit a down-the-line

shot and pass the net-player. This drill should be done to the forehand and backhand sides of the baseline player.

2. *Cross-Court Passing Shot.* With the same up-and-back alignment as in Drill 1, the baseline player hits to the net-player, who hits a deep corner. The baseline player tries to pass the net-player with a cross-court shot. This drill should be done to the forehand and backhand sides of the baseline player.

3. *Two Up, One Back Passing Shot.* The net-player makes the baseline player run back and forth, up and back. This drill provides practice on all the possible shots necessary in a game and is an outstanding conditioner.

12 Doubles Play Strategy

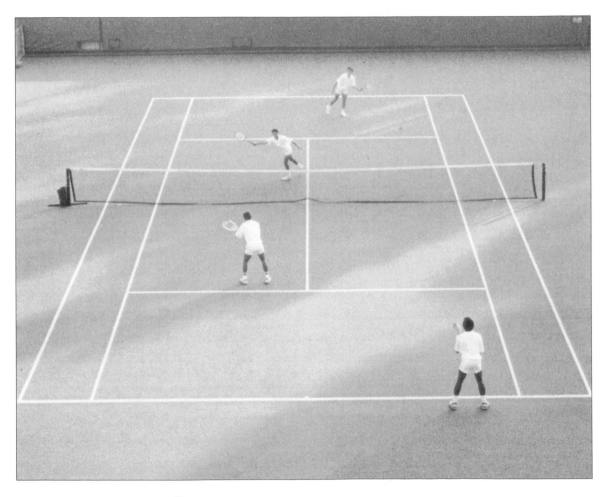

Outline

In doubles play, each player has less court to defend than is necessary in singles. In singles play, the player has 27 feet of width, compared with only 18 feet in doubles (the doubles court is 36 feet wide, and each player defends half of it). Because of this lessened area, players can attack more, which makes doubles play much more aggressive than singles. You don't just rally from the back court; you go after your opponents by playing the net.

Beginning Play

As in singles, the teams spin a racket to decide on whether the winning team will take "side or serve." Usually the winner will take the serve, so the losers get the better side.

The receiving team decides which player will receive on the forehand side (the deuce court) and which will take the serves to the backhand side (the ad court). Once this is decided, they must continue to receive serves in these positions throughout the set. They can change sides starting the next set, however.

The choice of receiving courts is often determined by who has the better backhand. The stronger backhand player will usually play the backhand court, the ad court. If one player is left-handed, that player may choose to play the ad court so that any wide serves will go to his or her forehand. With this arrangement, both players will have their forehands to the wide sides of the court. Another consideration could be to have the stronger player play the deuce court. So the choice of courts to defend is a highly individual choice depending on each player's strengths and those of your opponents.

The Serve

Once the serve is hit and returned, either player can hit any ball. Players are no longer restricted to playing one side of the court. The server serves first from the right court, just as in singles. The second point is served from the left, or ad, court. The server serves for the whole game. The serving court is the same as in singles. The 4 ½ foot alleys are not in bounds for serves.

In doubles it is even more important than in singles to get the first serve into the court. Since each player has less area to defend, and the service return is generally a weaker shot for most people, the serving team has a great advantage. So servers seldom try to ace their opponents but are content to use a lot of spin-serves. Good players usually try to get seven of every ten first serves in play.

Generally, you should hit your serve down the middle. This reduces the returner's angle and makes it easier for your partner, who is playing at the net, to try to cut off the receiver's return shot—by coming to the middle of the court (called *poaching*).

Sometimes you will want to get your opponent wide on the serve, so you spin-serve to make the ball bounce extra wide. A slice-serve to the deuce (opponent's right) court or a twist to the ad (left) court will serve to increase the area that the receiver has to cover. Such a wide serve will keep the receiver from aggressively coming to the net, because he or she will have to run wide and won't be able to run forward. This makes it very difficult, however, for your partner to poach.

When you serve down the middle to the deuce court, to your opponent's backhand, your partner will have a better chance to poach, because the receiver won't be able to hit the alley as well. So your partner should know where you intend to place your serve.

Although you will most often serve to your opponent's backhand, there are times when you will want to serve to the forehand side. Some people try to hit a full ground stroke on a service return and, consequently, often hit long. This type of player is a prime candidate to receive a forehand serve. Also, there are times when you can crowd a forehand, such as when serving a slice that starts at the backhand but spins toward the forehand.

Positioning

Since doubles is a game of attacking, both teams want to get to the net and attack their opponents. The server will serve from about halfway between the center mark and the sideline and will follow the spin-serve to the net.

The server's partner will already be at the net. The basic position is about halfway between the net and the service line—about 10 feet back from the net and a foot or two from the alley. From this position, the server's partner should

First serve alignment: Receivers deep

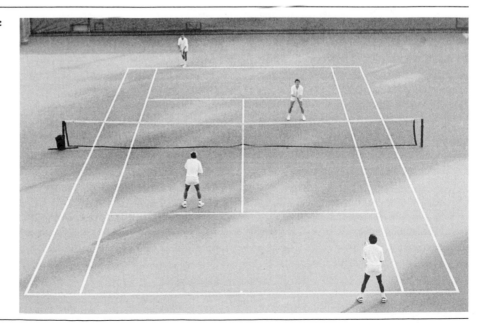

**Receiver moves up
for second serve**

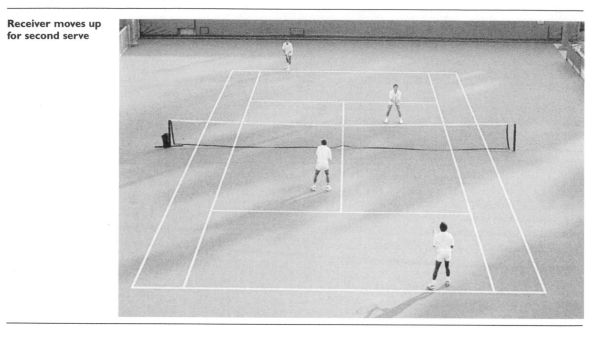

be prepared to hit any return of serve that can be reached. And sometimes he
or she will poach by running toward the other sidelines, trying to pick off the
return. But beware of poaching too often, because it may entice your opponent
to put one down the line for an easy point.

**Australian doubles
service alignment**

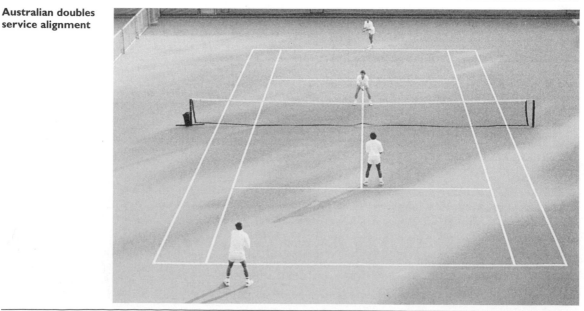

Australian doubles: Net player poaching and server moving to the backhand court

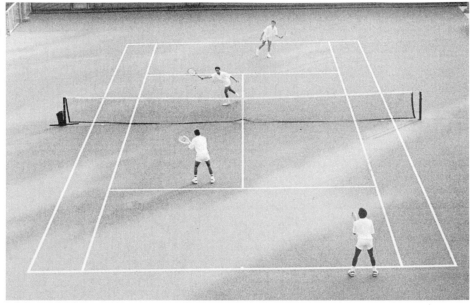

In one type of service strategy, called *Australian doubles*, the net-player stands in front of the server rather than on the other side. The net-player signals which direction he or she will go after the serve, and the server will then take the other side. This is quite unnerving for the receiving team, which can't be certain that the normal cross-court return will be open but must prepare for the possibility of going right back to the net-player. This is generally a better strategy for a first serve than for a second.

The Receiver

The receiver will play a bit wider in doubles than in singles, because the server in doubles has a wider angle to hit. The width depends on the angle that the server has in hitting the service court. Most players will play just inside the singles out-of-bounds line.

The receiver's partner will start at the service line so that if the net-player on the other team intercepts the return of service, it can't be put down the middle of the court. This is also a perfect place for calling the "out" serves. From this spot, it is easy to move forward to a good net position or to move to the back court.

The receiving team will also try to get to the net together. But it will be more difficult for them to get to the net on a service return than for the servers following their stronger shot. And while some receivers are able to take the net on a return, the major objective of the service return is to get the ball in play.

The server and receiver are wider in doubles than in singles

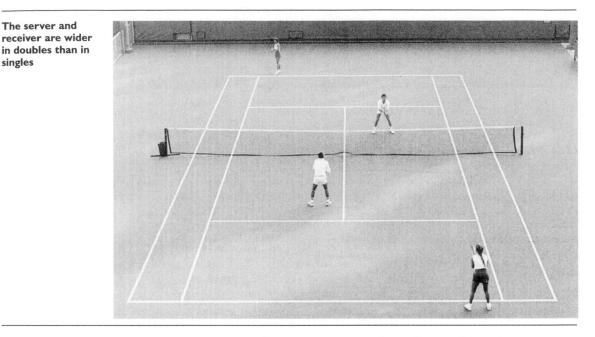

Most returns are made cross-court, away from the net-player. But sometimes you will want to lob your return safely over the net-player—especially if that player likes to poach a lot.

During the rally, both players want to be playing side by side—either both up at the net or both behind the baseline—as soon as possible. The net is much preferred.

Both receivers back in alignment

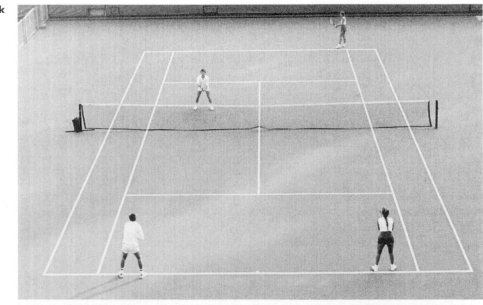

Beginners often play one up and one back while rallying. This gives far too many angles for the other team to hit, since the area open between these players and the area in front of the deeper player is wide open. It is quite acceptable for both players on the receiving team to start at the baseline rather than one up and one back. Furthermore, this alignment works well against a poaching team. It also works when the receivers keep the ball away from the net-player who is the stronger player on the team. It is a good strategy as well when one of your opponents is significantly weaker. This strategy is also often effective against the Australian doubles strategy.

Against the Australian doubles alignment, your return should be down the alley, since your opponents are both starting in the middle of their court. A lob return can also be effective.

Cross-Court Rally

The cross-court rally begins with the serve and return of serve. Both deep players try to keep the balls away from the players at the net. And each deep player tries to find an opening to get to the net. So the objective of the cross-court rally is to keep the opponent's deep player behind the baseline and to take advantage of any short shot to make an approach to the net.

During this deep rally, the net players slide towards the direction of the ball. Each is responsible for covering his or her half of the court; therefore, when the ball is on the other side of the net, the net-player should be approximately between the ball and the center of his or her half of the baseline.

In doubles, the objective from the back court is to keep the ball in play and let your opponents make a mistake. So the serve must be more consistent than in singles, and the ground strokes must be higher and more accurately placed.

Playing at the Net

You can attack at the net. From the net positions, you have much greater angles in which to hit your shots, and your shots will reach your opponents more quickly so they won't have time to make calculated shots. Moreover, you can often hit down at the ball and thus reduce your margin of error.

In advanced tennis, when both partners are at the net, they will play about 10 to 15 feet back from the net. From this spot they are in good position to volley and still be able to cover lobs. Beginners will usually play closer to the net so that they can volley more easily, but they are sitting ducks for an effective lob.

Both players should watch the ball at all times, except the net-player when his or her partner is serving. When you see your partner's shot, it gives you a better idea as to which way to move to better defend your opponent's return shot.

Volleys should usually be hit down the middle so that your opponents have a reduced angle for their return shot. It is generally understood that the player with the forehand will play most of the shots down the middle.

Keep your shots low to make your opponents hit up on the ball. Then you will be able to hit down on it for a winner. A good place to aim is at the feet of the opponent who is the closest to you.

When there is a doubt as to which player will take the shot, such as a lob, one of the players should call "mine" to alert his or her partner. And when one player has to take a shot in the other player's half of the court, they should switch. It is best to yell "switch" when you are sure you want to change sides. This is often done when a baseline player goes behind the net-player for a lob. Or it can be called by the net-player when he or she knows that the lob can't be reached.

If your team is forced to lob a ball, both players should hustle to the back court in order to defend against the overhead smash that will probably be your opponents' answer to your lob.

Poaching

A net-player may poach any time it seems likely that the receiver's return can be hit. This may occur on a service return or any time during the cross-court rally. It is more likely to be effective on a first serve. It can also help you out of trouble if you are behind, especially when your opponents have the ad. Since they will be thinking of a conservative cross-court return, you must think of an aggressive poach.

In poaching, the net player moves diagonally forward so that the hit can be made closer to the net. The point of aim is the open area of the court between the opponents or at the feet or hip of the opposing net-player.

Poaching: Net-player crosses to right court while server covers left court

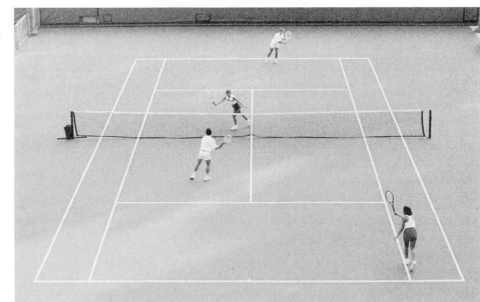

> ### ✓ Checklist for Doubles Play Strategy
>
> 1. Know and understand your partner.
> 2. Help to make your partner a better player.
> 3. Keep communicating with your partner throughout the match.
> 4. Keep the ball down the middle.
> 5. Get in a high percentage of first serves.
> 6. If your partner is at the net, you must take the offensive with your returns.
> 7. Call out "mine" when you can hit the ball. Rarely call "yours."

Signaling your serving partner of your intention to poach will make the server's positioning more effective by taking the doubt out of where you will be. You might use a hand signal behind your back, with a fist meaning that you will poach, one finger meaning you will stay, and two fingers meaning that you will fake a poach but stay.

The situation, rather than a prearranged poach, may dictate when you leave your net "home base." A softer or higher than normal shot may be a signal to go for it. A deep shot by your partner may also give you the opportunity to poach for a winner.

Poaching makes your opponents think. And the more you get athletes thinking, rather than reacting, the less effective they will be.

Getting to the Net

Getting to the net first is essential in controlling the game. And the team that gets to the net first will usually win the point. Following a first serve, which is usually deeper, is a common tactic. Following the second serve is not as common, because it is usually a safer serve and so will land shorter, giving the receiver a chance to come in on it and hit a powerful shot. In fact, the short serve is more likely to allow the receiver, rather than the server, to come to the net.

Once the rally has begun, with one player up and one back, the back court player looks for a short return on which to make the approach to the net. Any shot landing near the service line is a great opportunity to come to the net.

In advanced doubles, the server comes to the net on both the first and second serve.

Summary

1. In doubles, it is important to keep the ball in play and let your opponents make the mistake.
2. The advantage goes to the team that gets to the net first.

3. The players should stay side to side if at all possible—both at the net or both back.

4. Communicate with your partner. Yell "mine" or "yours" on doubtful shots, yell "switch" when one player crosses the court to get a shot, and signal where the serve will be or whether the net-player will poach or stay.

5. It is very important to get the first serve in play.

6. The server will generally serve from a wider position than in singles. The width of the server's position dictates the width of the receiver's position.

7. The server serves from the same court as in singles—even-numbered points from the deuce court and odd-numbered points from the ad court.

8. The receivers will defend the same court (ad or deuce) throughout the set.

9. Generally serve down the middle of the court.

10. Australian doubles service has both players in the middle of the court. It is often a good strategy for first serves.

Drills for Players at All Levels

These drills are discussed further and illustrated in Chapter 14.

1. *Positioning.* With one team up and one back, rally the ball. The up team must concentrate on moving with the ball and protecting the middle of the baseline on their half of the court. By staying between the ball and the middle of their half of the baseline, the players will cut down the angles that their opponents would otherwise have.

2. *Playing the Lob.* The baseline team rallies, then one hits a lob over the heads of the net-team. The net-team members both move back. One will call for the ball. If a crossing action is needed, one will yell "switch."

3. *Poaching* is practiced with a back court hitter drop-serving a cross-court shot, and the net-player crossing diagonally forward to intercept the ball.

4. *Serve.* With one player on each side of the net, the server hits a serve, hits an approach shot, then comes to the net.

13 *Taking Care of Your Mind and Body*

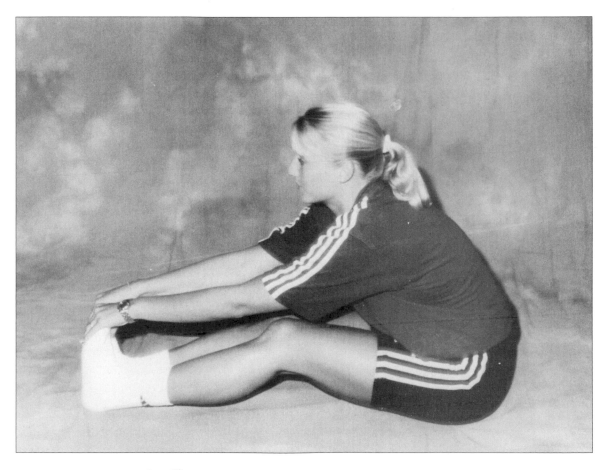

Outline

Wishing won't make you a better player; you must practice. Your practice can take place on the court, learning the physical skills of tennis; and it can also take place in a gym, conditioning your body. It can even take place at home, just mentally practicing. There are so many skills to practice in tennis, and there are so many ways to practice them, that you should always be able to help your game in some way.

Mental Practice

Championship athletes have known for years that mental practice helps their coordination. Only recently have sports psychologists refined the methods of perfecting the mind's contribution to the game.

Mental Imagery

The name for mental practice is *mental imagery*. It can be accomplished from the outside, such as by watching tennis on a videotape or by imagining seeing yourself practicing perfect form. For his sport, the golfer Jack Nicklaus calls this "going to the movies." In a second type of mental imagery, you are the "star" in your movie. You close you eyes and feel yourself in motion.

When you are mentally experiencing your game, you can practice your strokes and footwork or your strategy. In fact, you can practice whatever is giving you trouble. What if your service return is a problem. Just imagine yourself ready for the return. Your imaginary opponent tosses the ball and serves to your backhand. You feel yourself moving left and starting your backswing. You watch the ball. As you step and start your swing, you are always watching the ball. You complete your swing, still watching the ball.

Relaxation

Another essential of good tennis is relaxation. When you are relaxed, you can react more quickly to the ball. You can practice breathing deeply before you are ready to serve or receive.

Concentration

Concentration is the third major area of mental practice. The most important thing on which to concentrate is the ball. Not watching the ball all the way to your racket and while it is on your racket is probably the most common and critical error at every level of tennis. Slow-motion movies show us that most people take their eyes off the ball when it is still 4 to 6 feet away from them. They start looking at where they are going to hit it rather than watching the hit.

You should concentrate on seeing the spin of the ball, even the fuzz on the ball, as it comes to you. Watch it on your racket. Then continue to watch the spot where you hit the ball, even after the ball has left your racket.

Physical Conditioning

Strength

Strength is essential for most athletic events. In tennis, leg strength is needed to move and to make every shot. Abdominal and shoulder strength are essential to move through the ball smoothly and effortlessly. And wrist strength is necessary for every shot. Maximum strength is gained by exhausting your muscles in a few repetitions.

Wrist strength, actually *forearm strength*, is essential in serving. About half of beginners don't have the necessary strength to swing the racket up and hammer the ball down toward the court. Also, many players get *tennis elbow* as a result of weak forearm muscles and tendons. To practice the serve, you should do wrist curls with weights. A simple way to gain forearm strength quickly is to simply hold the end of a broom, palm up, then raise the broom. You will generally have enough forearm strength to serve properly within a week of practicing this exercise daily.

Developing forearm strength for the serve using a broom

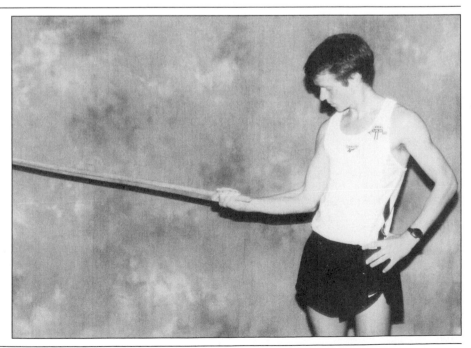

Developing back-of-wrist strength

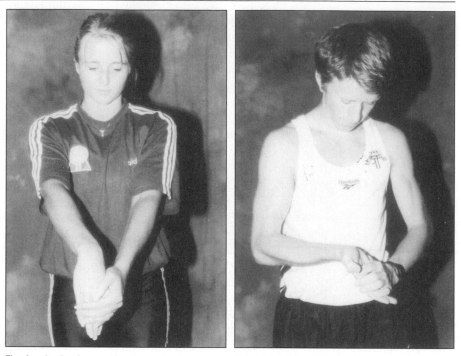

Flex hand palm down and resist   Extend one hand back at wrist and resist

You can develop the resistance-strength needed for the serve by bending one hand back at the wrist, then, with the other hand offering resistance, bringing the bent wrist through 180 degrees. Do the same exercise for the back of your forearm, palm down, to help strengthen your forearm for your backhand. Resistance-strength can also be developed by pushing against the back of your hand and making it work through a full range of motion.

Squeezing a ball or a grip strengthener is great for developing stronger hands and forearms.

Triceps strength is needed to bring the racket up in the serve. The triceps are weak in most people, so additional strength can help you to bring the racket up quickly and to either hit through the ball on a flat serve or to add extra spin on a slice serve. Pullovers or working with pulleys are good triceps exercises. Or you can take that same broom, hold it at the end, and with your elbow up like a serve, serve with the broomstick—not too fast!

To develop triceps strength with manual resistance, bend your right arm by touching your shoulder with your hand. Now take the other hand and place it against the wrist of your bent arm. Straighten your arm as you give yourself resistance.

**Developing triceps
strength**

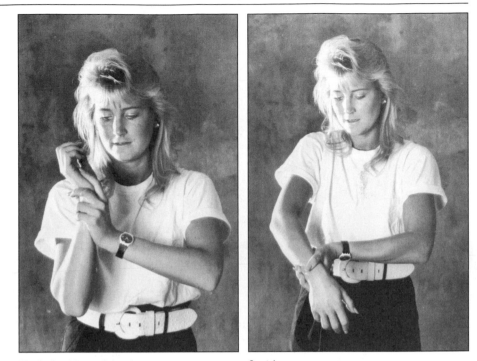

Touch shoulder with hand   Straighten arm

Upper-back muscles are used in hitting the backhand. If you have dumbbells, take one in each hand, bend over, and lift the dumbbells up to your side.

Leg power can be developed by simply jumping. Or if you have access to weights or a gym, do leg extensions, presses, or half-squats.

Back extensions are done on a Roman chair. Bend forward, then raise straight back. This exercise can also be done on the floor. Lie on the floor face down and, arching up just a little, slightly lift your shoulders and knees just off the floor. Don't lift your chest and knees more than two inches off the floor. (If you arch up too high, it is called *hyperextension*, and this is not a recommended exercise.) These lower back muscles are often injured in everyday activities, so this exercise should be done throughout your life.

Abdominal muscles are best strengthened with abdominal curl-ups. With your knees bent and your back on the floor, curl forward, keeping your hips (belt) on the ground. This is another good lifelong exercise.

The *inner and outer parts of your hips* can be strengthened on a special hip machine, if one is available. Otherwise, the following exercise can be done with a partner. Lie on your back with your legs in the air, and have your partner grasp your ankles. Push your legs out with the partner resisting. Then pull your legs in with your partner again resisting.

Flexibility

You need good flexibility throughout your body in order to move smoothly through a full range of motion in every stroke and serve. These flexibility exercises may be done after you have warmed up before every practice and before every match. They not only make you more flexible, but they get your muscles more ready to play. If you need more flexibility, for example in your calf muscle, stretch after practice and stretch farther, holding the stretches longer. Stretching when you are very warm is more likely to result in greater permanent flexibility.

The *upper chest* is stretched by bringing your arms to shoulder level, then pulling them backward as far as they will go.

For the *upper back*, bring them forward as far as possible and cross them.

For the *rear of the thighs*, slowly bend forward while sitting and touch your toes. If it is done standing, be sure to bend your knees slightly.

Groin area muscles are stretched by spreading your feet about 3 feet, bending your legs, then moving your torso over one leg, then the other.

Calf muscles are stretched by standing with your toes on a raised board, then letting the heels lower to the floor. It can also be done by standing 3 or 4 feet from a wall or fence and leaning on the support. With your legs straight and heels on the ground, drop your hips lower until you feel the stretch. Do every stretch slowly and for at least 20 seconds.

Abdominal muscles are stretched by slowly bending sideways.

The *back of the serving arm* can be stretched by pulling it across your chest with the other arm, or by holding it straight up and then applying pressure to the extended elbow from the outside in.

Back extensions exercise on Roman chair

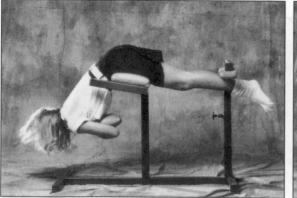

Bend at the waist   Straighten body

Chest stretch

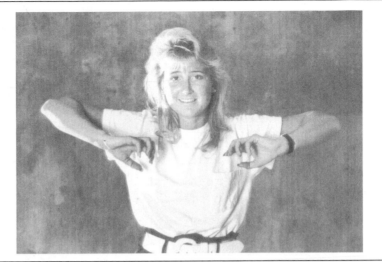

Aerobic (Cardiopulmonary) Conditioning

To develop your heart's ability to deliver oxygen to your muscles, you need to get your heart beating fast for a long time. The absolute minimum to make any improvement is 6 minutes, and for proper conditioning, you should work for at least 20 to 30 minutes with your heart rate at the *target level*.

The traditional method of determining your target heart rate is to merely subtract your age from the number 220, then working out with your pulse rate at a level of 65 to 90 percent of that number. For example, suppose you are 20 years old: 220 minus 20 equals 200, and a target rate of 65 percent would be 130 heart beats per minute, while a target rate of 85 percent would be 170 beats per minute. See the box on page 167 outlining Karvonen's more complicated, and more commonly accepted, method.

Any manner in which you can reach that level is acceptable. You can run, skip rope, cycle, or play continuous tennis (in which you keep running—you run while you rally, you run to pick up a ball, and you run back to the baseline). You can also condition yourself aerobically by playing imaginary tennis. Play against an imaginary partner with no ball. Practice your footwork, your approach shots, and your volley.

Common Injuries and How to Avoid Them

The facts about tennis—that it is generally played on a hard surface, while hitting a ball that is often moving quite fast, with a racket extending the arm and transferring significant force to the elbow and shoulder—give the sport some potentials for injury. The most common injuries are called ''overuse'' injuries

Stretching exercises

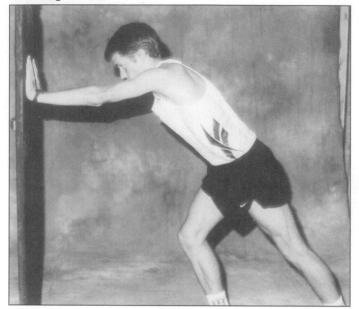

Calf stretch

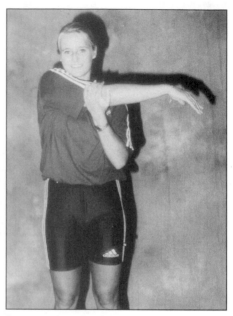

Stretching the back of the serving arm

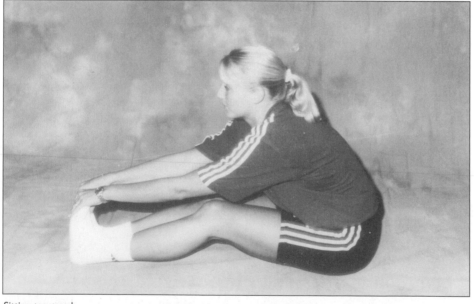

Sitting toe touch

because they occur over time after weeks, months, or years of strains on the muscles, tendons, and bones.

Elbow

The chronically stressed elbow can have muscular, tendon, or bursa damage and is seen in *tennis elbow*, in another type of tendinosis such as *Little League elbow*, or in a softened or damaged cartilage (chondromalacia). The sudden or acute type of injury can be a rupture of one of the elbow ligaments in a single throwing or serving action after many throws or serves have already stressed and weakened the ligament.

Tennis elbow (lateral humeral epicondylitis) can affect anyone who places continued strain on the back of the forearm. It is most common on the outside of the arm just under the elbow. It is caused primarily by hitting backhand shots. The muscles in the back of the forearm are not as strong as those on the inner side of the forearm, so they are more likely to be injured. This type of tennis elbow is most frequently found in recreational players.

You can also have a tennis elbow problem on the inside of the elbow. This is most likely caused by hitting hard serves and overheads, but continued hard forehand drives also contribute to the problem. The problem of tennis elbow on the inside (medial) part of the elbow is more common among elite players. This type of tennis elbow (medial epicondylitis) is also found in other athletes and may be called *golfer's elbow* or *pitcher's elbow*, depending on the sport. It is an inflammation of the tendons on the inside of the elbow caused by the straightening (extending) of the arm.

Tennis elbow problems occur in more than 40 percent (some estimate as high as 50 percent) of recreational tennis players over 30 years of age. Vibrations from the racket are a primary cause of the repeated stress to the forearm muscles and the elbow. When the ball is hit, vibrations develop. The farther from the sweet spot that you hit the ball, the greater the vibrations. Therefore, beginners are much more likely to incur elbow problems in tennis. Their muscles are not conditioned to the sport, and their coordination is not good enough yet to hit the ball in the middle of the racket on every stroke.

What to do:

1. R.I.C.E. (Rest, ice, compression, elevation).
2. Wear an elbow brace specifically designed for the condition. Most sporting goods stores and tennis shops stock them.
3. To prevent a recurrence, or to prevent it from happening in the first place, do wrist extension exercises. A reduced-vibration racket, such as a titanium racket, may help.

Tendon and muscle problems in the elbow can be prevented if the muscles around the elbow are strengthened so that they absorb more of the shock. For example, to prevent a tennis elbow, you should do reverse wrist curls or, more simply, just grasp the end of broom and, with your palm facing down, lift the broom using only the movement of the wrist. Do this several times each day to strengthen the muscles on the back side of the forearm. This strengthens the arm for backhand drives. To prevent the tennis elbow problems that occur on the inside of the forearm, lift the same broom with the palm of your hand facing upward. Use only wrist movement. This will also help you to develop strength for the serve.

Back

Chronic low back pain is a common complaint of more skilled tennis players. Nearly 40 percent of professional players have complained of this problem and have missed tournaments because of it. It can be caused by a number of factors. Tight buttock and hamstring muscles, tight connective tissue in the lower back, poor abdominal strength, poor posture (swayback), and muscle strains are the most common causes. The tennis serve is often a cause because the back is arched and is twisted with great force while it is arched. This can cause excessive stress on the lumbar disks.

Knees

Knee pain can affect every aspect of the knee. Pain in the front of the knee, or *housemaid's knee* (prepatellar bursitis), can be caused by such injuries as damage to the patellar tendon or an inflamed bursa (lubricating sac). It can be caused by continued trauma to the area or by a weakness of the hamstrings when compared with the quadriceps, which puts additional pressure on the front of the knee.

Damage to the back surface of the kneecap (patella) is medically termed chondromalachia patella (injury to the back of the kneecap) or patelliofemoral pain syndrome, but is commonly called "cyclist's knee" or "runner's knee." It has many causes, including the misalignment of the kneecap caused by a lack of flexibility, muscular weakness in the quadriceps, bone deformity, or a roughening of the smooth cartilage lining of the patella, which prevents it from riding smoothly in its most desired track.

Patellar tendinitis is common at all ages among runners, jumpers ("jumper's knee"), and tennis players. The continued flexion and extension of the knee joint during running can cause minute damages to the tendon. In more severe cases, the tendon can tear in the area of the patella or closer to the tendon's attachment below the knee.

Feet

When too much friction is put on the skin, it heats the skin and acts like a burn. This causes a *blister*. Blisters are produced when the skin is rubbed, and the outer layer of skin separates from the inner layer. Fluid from the second layer fills that separation. The more friction and the more heat produced, the larger the blister. The fluid inside the blister causes pain.

Blisters are most common on the back of the heel, on the toes, or under the ball of the foot. Stiff-heeled shoes, or shoes not properly laced, or shoes too big, or too small, or new, are often the cause of a blister. Blisters are far more likely at the beginning of a sport season. It is always a good idea to wear two pairs of thin socks when breaking in new shoes. The extra sock absorbs some of the rubbing that the skin would otherwise have to endure. If you notice a special pressure when you are active, paint the area that feels irritated with tincture of benzoine ("Tuff Skin"), then cover that with a cream or gel such as Vaseline.

What to do if you get a blister:

1. Use a donut-shaped pad around the blister to eliminate any more pressure.
2. Use a skin lubricant, such as Vaseline, over the blister to protect from any additional stress.
3. Keep the area clean because the blister may pop on its own and you do not want to invite infection.

To prevent blisters:

1. File down any calluses so blisters do not develop under them.
2. Always wear socks when you are wearing shoes.
3. Use two pairs of socks, especially early in the sport season.
4. Buy shoes with a proper fit and break in new shoes gradually.

Plantar fasciitis is a common complaint, especially with older athletes. It is said to affect nearly 20 percent of runners. The soreness is under the foot and in the heel or just forward of the heel. "Plantar" means the bottom of the foot, "fascia" is the connective tissue (tendons and ligaments), and "itis" means inflammation. It is usually caused by bruising of the tissue on or near the heel. The condition is generally a stress injury where the tendons under the foot are repeatedly stressed, such as in running in tennis.

Plantar fasciitis may occur in several tissues in the bottom of the foot. The most common area is on or just in front of the heel bone (calcaneus). The ligaments and tendons that attach to the heel are prone to problems from either trauma, overstretching, or tightening due to not being stretched often enough. Tight calf muscles and tendons (gastrocnemius and soleus) are often related to the cause, so stretching of the heel is always recommended as part of the cure. Stretching of the rear calf muscles should be done several times a day. The muscles that move the bones of the foot may also be bruised or stretched.

Another related cause is often that the foot is pronated (the inside part of the foot is closer to the ground). When this is the case, a proper orthotic device that lifts the long arch of the foot may both heal the foot and prevent a recurrence. The orthotic may take up to six months to cure the problem.

The pain is particularly noticeable when getting out of bed in the morning. It may also be evident when arising after being seated for some time. Rest is the major type of treatment. A donut pad or a rubber heel cup with extra cushioning underneath may also be an aid. Arch supports, which are made for increasing the arch of the foot, can also help.

Arch problems affect many people. There are two arches in the foot. One is under the base of the toes (the transverse arch) and the other runs from the front of the heel to the base of the toes (the metatarsal arch). These arches act as shock absorbers. Extra high or very low arches sometimes cause problems.

An orthotic inserted under a low arch will bring the foot closer to normal and will generally relieve any pain.

Very high arches may also cause problems, but an orthotic can give support. If the high arch is caused by tight connective tissue (ligaments and tendons) under the foot, hammertoes or plantar fasciitis may result.

Orthotic Devices

Orthotics are shoe inserts that generally affect the heel and both arches of the foot. Properly designed, they reduce foot, ankle, and lower leg problems. They are valuable in preventing or healing plantar fasciitis, shin splints, fallen or weak arches, and a number of other problems. Tennis players have found them to be helpful in holding the foot in its proper position and in making their shoes fit more effectively. Medical doctors, podiatrists, and chiropractors can all fit you for orthotics. You can purchase some orthotics that may work for you from sporting goods stores. They are made for the traditional problems in feet and may or may not work perfectly for you.

Heel cups can reduce or prevent some problems. The hard plastic heel cups can make up for poorly fitting heels in your shoes. The soft rubber heel cups can absorb shocks and help to prevent or ease those problems caused by continued stresses. Heel spurs, plantar fasciitis, and shin splints can be aided by rubber heel cups.

Summary

1. The complete tennis player must make use of his or her maximum mental and physical potentials. There are proven ways to improve one's tennis off the court.
2. Mental conditioning includes:
   - Imagery, in which you visualize the techniques and the game situations that may be encountered.
   - Relaxation, in which you dissipate tension and thus are able to perform at a higher level.
   - Concentration, in which you focus on a certain aspect of the game. A beginner might concentrate on the backswing or follow-through, while an intermediate or advanced player might concentrate on watching the ball.
3. Physical conditioning requires that the tennis player develop strength, flexibility, and cardiopulmonary endurance.
4. For a tennis player, strength and flexibility are most important in the thighs, groin, upper chest, back, triceps, forearms, and abdominals.
5. Proper stretching exercises not only prepare the muscles to react to their maximum potential, but also reduce the chances of muscular and connective tissue injuries.
6. Proper conditioning and equipment can reduce the chance of injury.

The Karvonen Formula

The Finnish scientist M. J. Karvonen has improved on the simple formula of 220 minus your age as the maximum heart rate. He starts with that number, but then subtracts the resting pulse rate to determine the "heart rate reserve."

1. First take 220 minus your age ____. This is your maximum heart rate (MHR).

   Next, determine your resting heart rate while lying in bed in the morning before you get up. Use your index and middle fingers and locate your pulse, either on the side of your neck (carotid artery) or on the wrist just above the thumb. Count the number of pulse beats in a minute, or take your pulse for 15 seconds and multiply by 4 to determine the total for a minute.

2. Resting heart rate (pulse rate) (rest HR) ____

3. Subtract your resting heart rate from the maximum pulse rate.

   MHR ____ - rest HR ____ = ____ heart rate reserve (HRR)

   Now you will determine your maximum and minimum pulse rates for an effective workout. For the average person, your high end will be your heart rate reserve multiplied by 80 percent (.80) added to your resting pulse rate.

4. ____(HRR) × .80 = ____ + ____ (rest HR) = ____ maximum desirable heart rate during exercise.

   Next find the minimal acceptable level for your workout by multiplying your heart rate reserve (HRR) by 60 percent (.60), added to your resting pulse rate.

5. ____ (HRR) × .60 = ____ + ____ (rest HR)=____ minimal desirable heart rate during exercise.

   These two percentages (60 and 80 percent) are not set in stone. If you have medical problems or are in very poor condition, you might use a number between 40 and 55 percent to set your minimal pulse rate. If you are very fit or a competitive athlete, you might use 85 or 90 percent to set your high-end exercise pulse rate.

   Here is an example of how a 20-year-old would determine her target training pulse range. Assume that her resting pulse rate is 70.

   Minimum target heart rate (220 - 20 = 200 - 70 = 130) × .60 = 78 + 70 = 148

   Maximum target heart rate (220 - 20 = 200 - 70 = 130) × .80 =104 + 70 = 174

   For a 40-year-old with a resting pulse of 65, the target heart rates would be:

   Minimum target heart rate (220 - 40 = 180 - 65 = 115) × .60 = 69 + 65 = 134

   Maximum target heart rate (220 - 40 = 180 - 65 = 115) × .80 = 92 + 65 = 157

14 *Practicing Effectively*

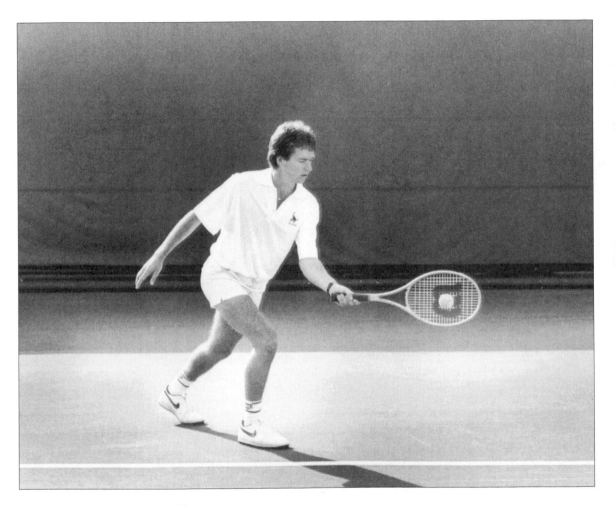

Outline

Drills for the Beginner
Drills for the Advanced Beginner to the Expert
Gamelike Drills
Doubles Drills
Warm-Up

As emphasized earlier, you cannot become a better player by wishing, but only by practice. However, more than that, the practice must be *effective* practice. In other words, "Practice doesn't make perfect—perfect practice makes perfect."

Since tennis is not an easy game to play, it takes years of practice to be truly proficient. Of course, you can have fun right from the beginning, but you will have more fun when the ball starts going where you want it and the way you want it. This takes confidence as well as skill, so effective practice should build your confidence.

With the exception of some very basic beginners' drills, the same drills can be used by the advanced beginner and the expert. Whether you are practicing a cross-court drill, a volley drill, or a lob and overhead drill, the same drill is suitable for every level of player. The difference is that the advanced and professional player will hit the ball harder and with more accuracy than the novice.

If a ball machine is available, it can be used by players of any skill level, simply by adjusting the velocity. Without a ball machine, beginners can practice by having a partner throw the ball to the correct spot so that it can be hit properly. As beginners improve, they can have their partner hit the ball to them. Intermediate players can rally with each other, putting the ball reasonably close to where they want it for the drill.

In each drill, have a target to hit. The better you become, the smaller the target area should be.

Drills for the Beginner

1. *Feeling the Ball on the Racket.* Hold the racket with your palm facing upward so that the flat part of the racket head is parallel to the ground. Place a ball on the sweet spot—the middle of the strings. Now just bounce the ball upward from the racket. How many times can you hit it upward without letting it hit the ground? Get used to feeling the ball bounce on your racket.

2. *Bounce the Ball on the Court.* Turn your palm so that it faces the ground. The racket head should be parallel to the ground. Now bounce the ball from the ground to your racket. How many times can you bounce it without missing?

   When you become proficient at bouncing the ball in one place, walk along and bounce the ball off the ground.

3. *Hitting Against "Air."* Practice the 1-2-3-4 count action described in the book for each stroke and serve. Practice your stroke without hitting a ball. You can practice this in front of a mirror at home. Get the feel of leaning into the ball as you hit it, and complete the full follow-through.

4. *Drop-Hit into a Fence.* With the racket in one hand and the ball in the other, drop the ball, then hit it into the fence after it has bounced off the ground.

5. *Hitting the Slow-Pitched Ball.* Using either a partner or a ball machine, have the ball pitched slowly to the hitting player. Let the ball bounce, then hit it.

6. *Hitting Against the Wall.* There are several drills in which a wall can be used:

   a. Standing about 25 feet from the wall, drop the ball and hit it to the wall, then catch it.

   b. Move farther away from the wall. Now hit and rally with yourself, keeping the ball in play as long as possible. Try to keep the ball between 4 and 7 feet from the ground. (Since the net is 3 to 3 ½ feet high, you must clear the net, but you should not hit the ball too high.)

   c. As you get better, move farther from the net, perhaps as far as 40 feet from the wall. You will have to get set more quickly, because the ball will return faster than it will when rallying with a partner. If you are 40 feet from the wall, the ball will travel 80 feet between each of your shots. On a court, the ball will travel about 160 feet (the length of the 78-foot court twice).

7. *The Toss Height.* Standing next to a fence or a wall, reach your racket as high as possible. If possible, mark the spot of the top of your racket. Now toss the ball to that spot. A perfect toss would be exactly at the middle of your racket (the sweet spot) at the top of its arc. By tossing to the top of your racket, you allow yourself a small margin of error.

8. *Placing the Toss.* Take your serving stance and place your racket on the ground with the head just ahead of your forward foot. Toss the ball to the proper height and let it drop to the ground. If it hits your racket head, it is placed perfectly.

9. *Serving into a Fence* allows the server to perfect the serving action without worrying about whether or not the ball will go into the service court.

10. *Serving from the Service Line* gives the server a much easier target to hit.

Drills for the Advanced Beginner to the Expert

On all drills for ground strokes, hit the ball deep. Try to get the ball within 5 feet of the baseline.

1. *Forehand Down-the-Line Shots* can be practiced with the help of a partner or a ball machine. The partner tosses or hits the ball to your forehand, and you hit the down-the-line shot. You can place a target inside the sideline and inside the back court line according to your skill level.

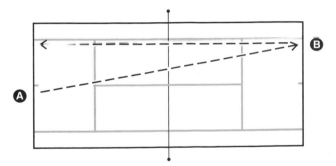

2. *Backhand Down-the-Line Shots* can be practiced the same way.

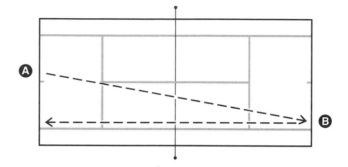

3. *Combination Ground Strokes*. One player hits a down-the-line forehand, the other player returns it down the line with a backhand. This is a drill for high-intermediate to advanced players. The drill should be done on one side of the court, then the other, so that each player has a chance to practice both the forehand and the backhand down-the-line shots.

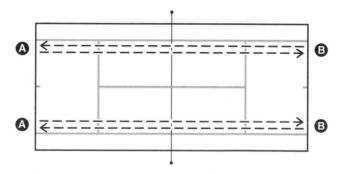

4. *Cross-Court Shots* are practiced the same way—forehand and backhand. For the best practice and for better physical conditioning, return to the center of your court after each shot.

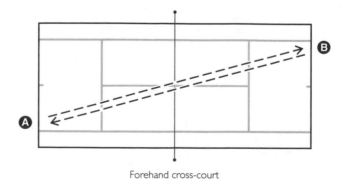

Forehand cross-court

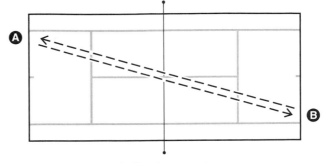

Backhand cross-court

5. *Combination Ground Stroke Drill* has one player hitting only cross-court shots and the other hitting only down the line. This drill forces both players to run and hit. It helps your conditioning as well as your stroke development.

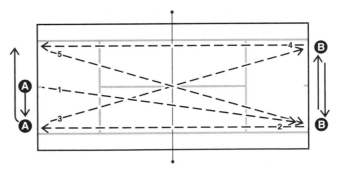

6. *Touch or Drop Shot.* With both players at the net, one feeds the other a straight shot, which is then hit with an accentuated slicing action so that it either stops or bounces back toward the net after it hits the ground. The drop-shotting player should almost catch the ball on the racket as the racket is cut sharply under the ball. You will need maximum spin and minimum speed on the ball as it barely clears the net. The advanced player will fake a hard shot before making the drop shot.

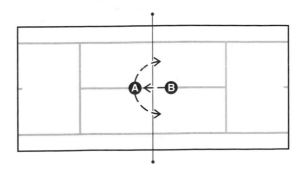

7. *Volleying* is best started with one player hitting to the forehand, then to the backhand of the volleyer. Later both players can volley easily—just hitting the ball, not trying to pass the opponent. Practice looking at the ball. As you progress, start aiming for the corners of the service court—to increase the angle that your opponent must cover.

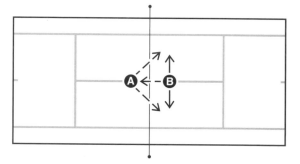

8. *Volleying Against the Wall* is a way to practice the volley without any help. Stand about 10 feet from the wall. First hit all forehand volleys, then all backhands, then alternate.

9. *One Up–One Back Rally.* This drill can be done forehand to forehand, backhand to backhand, or with a combination of shots. It can also be done with the net-player hitting directly to the baseline player, but the baseline player hitting shots from side to side for the volleyer.

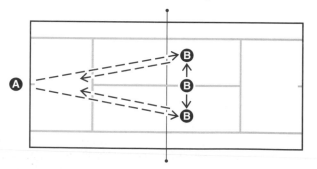

10. *Back Court-Volley Combination* is started as a back court rally. When your opponent hits a short shot, attack the ball, make an approach shot, then volley.

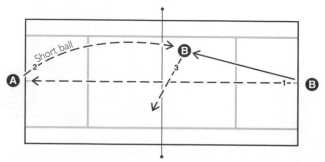

11. *Reflex Volley Drill* has both players at the net. Keep the ball in the air—don't let it bounce. Both players should start at the service line and move in one step after each hit. Hit each shot at your opponent or at your opponent's feet—don't try for a sideline shot. Hit the ball with some backspin by hitting down on it with the racket face a little open.

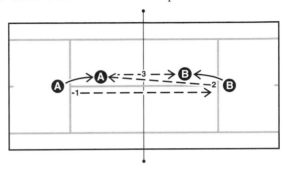

12. *Lobs* can be practiced with each player hitting to the other. Start with defensive (high) lobs, then work on the offensive (low) lobs.

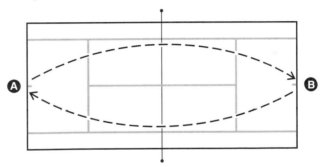

13. *Overhead Smashes* are best started with one player lobbing to the other, forcing the net-player to run back, get in position behind the ball, then smash it. The player hitting the overhead must return to the net after each smash, then move back to hit the next overhead.

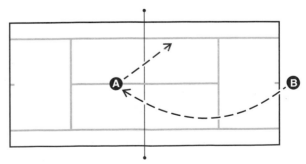

14. *Lob-Overhead Combination* is done with one player lobbing and the other hitting overheads. The person hitting the overhead must come to the net and touch it with the racket after the hit.

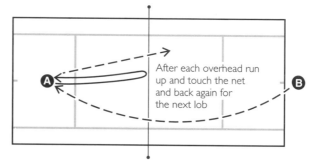

15. *Serving at Targets*. Place targets (tennis ball cans or cardboard) on the serving court. One target should be 3 feet short of the service line and along the boundary toward which you will aim your slice-serve. (For right-handed servers, it will be to the left of the court as you look at it.) A second target should be in the opposite corner of the service court. (For right-handed servers, it will be to your right in the service court—toward your right-handed opponent's backhand.) The third target should be directly where your opponent would stand. (For a right-handed opponent, it will be 3 to 4 feet in from the center line and just inside the service line.) This is called a jam serve.

   Practice serving at each target. You will get a thrill each time you knock over a ball can with a perfect serve.

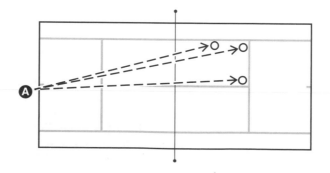

16. *Service Return*. Have a partner stand near the service line of the opposite court and serve you the ball. By being closer, your partner has a better chance of getting the ball in the court, and you will have to react faster to make your return.

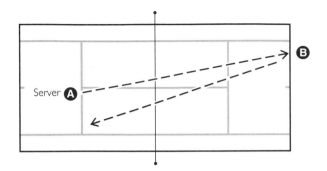

17. *Serve and Return* allows the players to practice the two most difficult aspects of the game and then play the point out.

Gamelike Drills

1. *Down-the-Line Passing Shots.* The baseline player hits to the net-player, who hits to a deep corner. The baseline player attempts to hit a down-the-line shot and pass the net-player. This drill should be done to the forehand and backhand sides of the baseline player.

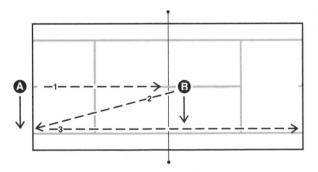

Passing shot—forehand

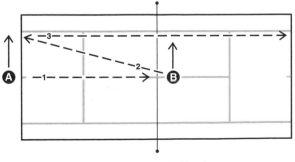

Passing shot—backhand

2. *Cross-Court Passing Shots.* With the same up-and-back alignment, the baseline player hits to the net-player, who hits a deep corner. The baseline player tries to pass the net-player with a cross-court shot. This drill should be done to the forehand and backhand sides of the baseline player.

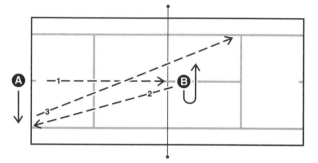

Cross-court passing shot—forehand

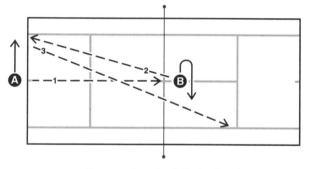

Cross-court passing shot—backhand

3. *Two Up–One Back Passing Shots.* The net-players make the baseline player run back and forth, up and back. This drill provides practice for all the possible shots in a game and is an outstanding conditioner.

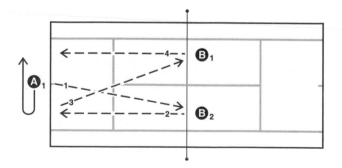

Doubles Drills

1. *Positioning.* With one team up and one back, rally the ball. The up team must concentrate on moving with the ball and protecting the middle of the baseline on their half of the court. By staying between the ball and the middle of their half of the baseline, the players will cut down the angles that their opponents would otherwise have.

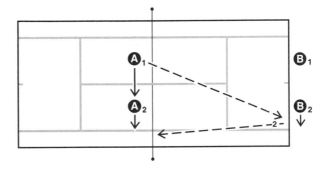

2. *Playing the Lob.* The baseline team rallies, then one of the players hits a lob over the heads of the net team. The net-team members both move back. One will call for the ball. If a crossing action is needed, one will yell "switch."

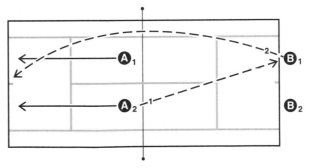

Playing the lob—drop back

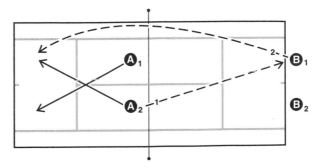

Playing the lob—drop and switch

3. *Poaching* is practiced with a back court player hitting a cross-court shot, and the net-player crossing diagonally forward to intercept the ball.

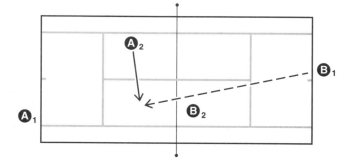

4. *Serve.* With one player on each side of the net, the server hits a serve, hits an approach shot, then comes to the net.

Warm-Up

An adequate warm-up is essential to get your muscles ready to react properly when you play and to reduce your chance of injury by straining a muscle.

Start by warming up with jumping jacks or a little jogging. You may want to do some stretching exercises explained in the previous chapter. (Recent research, however, indicates that stretching, at least for runners, may increase injuries.) On cooler days, take longer on this part of the warm-up.

In a warm-up before practice or a match, start at the baseline and softly rally the ball, watching it all the way into your racket. As you feel more confident, move back behind the baseline and continue the rally. As you practice each type of shot, always start slowly; then as you warm, hit harder.

Work with your partner on lobs and overheads. One should lob while the other smashes until each feels comfortable; then they should switch shots. Next, one should come to the net and volley while the other plays the back court. Later, they again switch. Finally, practice the serve and the return. On the return, concentrate on watching the ball come off the server's racket, and move to it. Practice as many serves and returns as you feel necessary, because you can't take practice serves once the match has begun.

15 *Nutrition for Better Conditioning*

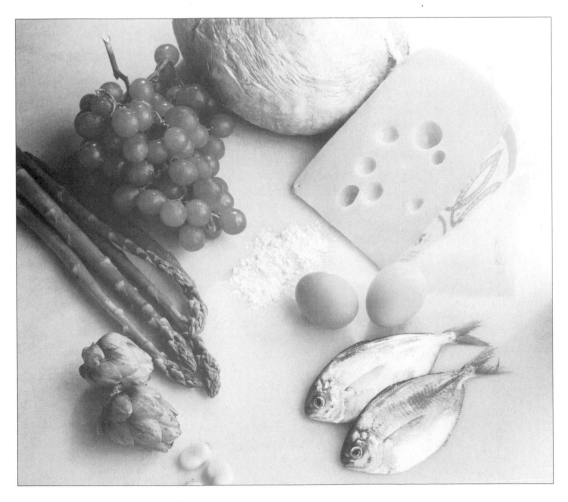

Outline

Along and full life requires exercise, an adequate diet, and play—both physical and mental—and a basic understanding of the science of nutrition is essential to healthy living. If you are going to play tennis you will need adequate fuel for your athletic body. This chapter describes the basic elements of good nutrition. In the next chapter we will discuss how to apply these nutritional principles to your diet and weight management.

Nutrition

An informed person is aware of the nutrients necessary for minimal function, and can then put that knowledge into practice by developing a proper diet. Unfortunately, very few people consume even the minimum amounts of each of the necessary nutrients—protein, fat, carbohydrates, vitamins, minerals, and water (the essential nonnutrient). The first three nutrients listed (protein, fat, and carbohydrates) provide the energy required to keep us alive, in addition to making other specific contributions to our bodies.

The calorie measure used in counting food energy is really a kilocalorie— one thousand times larger than the calorie used as a measurement of heat in your chemistry class. In one food calorie (kilocalorie), there is enough energy to heat one kilogram of water one degree Celsius, or to lift 3,000 pounds of weight one foot high. So those little calories you see listed on cookie packages pack a lot of energy.

Most people need about 10 calories per pound of body weight just to stay alive. If you plan to do something other than just lie in bed all day, you probably need about 17 calories per pound of body weight per day in order to keep yourself going. And if you decide to play a couple of hours of singles, you can count on using a whole lot more calories.

Protein

Protein is made up of 22 *amino acids*, which consist of carbon, hydrogen, oxygen, and nitrogen. While both fats and carbohydrates contain the first three elements, nitrogen is found only in protein. Protein is essential for building nearly every part of the body—the brain, heart, organs, skin, muscles, and even the blood.

There are four calories in one gram of protein. Adults require 0.75 grams of protein per kilogram of body weight per day; this translates into one-third a gram of protein per pound. So an easy way to estimate your protein requirements in grams per day would be to divide your body weight by three. For instance, if you weigh 150 pounds, you need about 50 grams of protein per day.

Physically active adults have been thought to require more protein than is recommended by the United States Recommended Daily Allowance (USRDA), which is set at .8 grams per kilogram of body weight per day. In fact, most active people do not need to eat additional protein if 12 to 15 percent of their total calories is protein. Since active individuals need to consume more calories per day than their inactive counterparts due to their increased energy expenditure, active adults who keep their protein intake at around 15 percent of their total calories will eat more protein per day and thereby fulfill their body's protein requirement. Excess protein consumption (above the body's requirement) is broken down and the calories are either burned off or stored as fat.

However, when you are involved in a strenuous strength training regimen, as you might be if you play competitive tennis, it may be necessary to increase your protein intake percentage, depending on the number of total calories you consume per day.

In order for your body to make any kind of tissue, including muscle, you must first have all of the necessary amino acids. Your body can manufacture some of them, while you must get others from your food. Those amino acids that you must get from your food are called the *essential amino acids*, while the others that you can make are known as the *nonessential amino acids*. During childhood, nine of the 22 amino acids are essential, while in adulthood we acquire the ability to synthesize one additional amino acid, leaving us with eight essential amino acids.

Amino acids cannot be stored in the body, so we need to consume our minimum amounts of protein every day. If adequate protein is not consumed, the body immediately begins to break down tissue (usually beginning with muscle tissue) to release the essential amino acids. If even one essential amino acid is lacking, the other essential ones are not able to work to their capacities. For example, if methionine (the most commonly lacking amino acid) is present at 60 percent of the minimum requirement, the other seven essential amino acids are limited to near 60 percent of their potential. When they are not used, amino acids are excreted in the urine.

Animal products (fish, poultry, and beef) and animal byproducts (milk, eggs, and cheese) are rich in readily usable protein. This means that when you eat animal products or by-products, the protein you consume can be converted into protein in your body because these sources have all of the essential amino acids in them. These foods are called *complete protein sources*.

Incomplete protein sources are any other food sources that provide protein but not all of the essential amino acids. Examples of incomplete proteins include peas and nuts. These food sources must be combined with other food sources that have the missing essential amino acids so that you can make protein in your body. Examples of complementary food combinations are rice and beans or peanut butter on whole wheat bread.

Another reason to be aware of complementary food combinations is that they enhance the absorption of the protein consumed. The person who is aware of the varying qualities of proteins can combine them to take advantage of the strengths of each. For example, if you eat flour at breakfast in the form of a piece of toast or coffee cake and wash it down with coffee, then drank a glass of milk at lunch, each of the protein sources would be absorbed by your body at a lower level. But if you ate bread with the milk at either meal, the higher protein values of both would be absorbed by your body immediately.

Fats

Fat is made of carbon, hydrogen, and oxygen. There are nine calories in a gram of fat. In the body, fat is used to develop the myelin sheath that surrounds the nerves. It also aids in the absorption of vitamins A, D, E, and K, which are the fat-soluble vitamins. It serves as a protective layer around our vital organs, and it is a great insulator against the cold. It is also a great concentrated energy source. And of course its most redeeming quality is that it adds flavor and juiciness to food!

Just as protein is broken down into different kinds of nitrogen compounds called amino acids, there are also different kinds of fats. There are three major kinds of fats, or fatty acids: saturated fats, monounsaturated fats, and polyunsaturated fats.

Saturated fats are "saturated" with hydrogen atoms. They are generally solid at room temperature and are most often found in animal fats, eggs, and whole milk products. Since these are the fats that are primarily responsible for raising the blood cholesterol level and hardening the arteries, they should be minimized in your diet.

Monounsaturated fats (oleic fatty acids) have room for two hydrogen ions to double-bond to one carbon. They are liquid at room temperature and are found in great amounts in olive, peanut, and canola (rapeseed) oils. Dietary monounsaturated fats have been shown to help the body excrete dietary cholesterol, thereby contributing a positive effect on atherosclerosis, one type of arteriosclerosis.

Polyunsaturated fats (linoleic fatty acids) have at least two carbon double bonds available, which translates into space for at least four hydrogen ions. Polyunsaturated fats are also liquid at room temperature and are found in the highest proportions in vegetable sources. Safflower, corn, and linseed oils are good sources of this type of fat. Polyunsaturated fatty acids of the omega-3 type may also contribute to the prevention of atherosclerosis.

We eat too much fat. The minimum requirement for fat in the diet is considered to be somewhere between 10 and 20 percent of the total calories consumed. The absolute maximum should be 30 percent, which is the amount now recommended for the American diet. While we as a society are still above this 30 percent value, we have been declining since the 1970s, and we need to keep that trend going. Most of us consume between 35 and 50 percent of our total calories in fats, with a very high percentage in saturated fats—the fats that we want to avoid.

Our high fat intake, most of which is saturated, tends to raise blood cholesterol levels in many people. If you are interested in decreasing the chances of developing hardened arteries by lowering your blood cholesterol level, it is recommended that you follow a diet low in fat (with the saturated fat intake at 10 percent or less of your total diet) and consume less than 300 milligrams of cholesterol daily. Or to put it another way, keep the total calories from fat under a third of your total intake and eat twice as much polyunsaturated and monounsaturated fat as saturated fat.

In the past, companies were allowed to identify the oil in a product on their labels as simply vegetable oil; under the Food and Drug Administration requirements made in 1976, they are now required to note whether it is corn oil, cottonseed oil, soybean oil, and so on, because some oils, even though they are not of animal origin, are very high in saturated fat. Palm kernel oil and coconut oil, often referred to as "tropical oils," are particularly high in saturated fats.

When you buy foods, especially cookies and crackers, always check the type of fat used. Avoid those with palm kernel oil and coconut oil. Also be aware of the hydrogenated oils used. While a hydrogenated safflower or canola oil may still have an acceptable fat ratio, a hydrogenated peanut or cottonseed oil may not contain the desired levels of unsaturated fats. Partially hydrogenated vegetable oils may contribute to the development of heart disease. The dietary use of hydrogenated corn oil stick margarine has been shown to increase LDL cholesterol levels when compared to the use of similar amounts of corn oil, also indicating an increased risk of heart disease.

In terms of controlling one's blood cholesterol level, dietary cholesterol is not as important as saturated fats in your diet. For this reason, saturated fats such as red meats, butter, egg yolks, chicken skin, and other animal fats should be greatly decreased. As an informed consumer, you may want to keep track of both your total fat intake and your intake of saturated fat to become better aware of your potential risk for heart disease. For example, one egg contains 5.6 grams of fat and only 0.7 grams of polyunsaturated fat, while an equal weight of hamburger contains 8.7 grams of fat and only 0.4 grams of polyunsaturated fats.

Carbohydrates

Carbohydrates are made from carbon, hydrogen, and oxygen, just as are fats, but "carbs" are generally a simpler type of molecule. There are four calories in a gram of carbohydrate. If carbohydrates are not utilized as immediately for energy as sugar (glucose), they are either stored in the body as glycogen (the stored form of glucose) or synthesized into fat and stored. Some carbohydrates cannot be broken down by the body's digestive processes; these are called fibers and will be discussed later. Digestible carbohydrates, can be separated into two categories: simple and complex. *Simple carbohydrates* are the most readily usable energy source in the body and include such things as sugar, honey, and fruit. *Complex carbohydrates* are the starches, which also break down into sugar for energy, but their breakdown is slower than with simple "carbs." Complex carbohydrates also bring with them various vitamins and minerals.

People in the United States often eat too many simple carbohydrates. These are often referred to as "empty calories," because they have no vitamins, minerals, or fibers. While a person who uses a great deal of energy can consume these empty calories without potential weight gain, most of us find these empty calories settling on our hips. The average person consumes 125 pounds of sugar per year, which is equivalent to one teaspoon every 40 minutes, night and day. Since each teaspoon of sugar contains 17 calories, this amounts to 231,000 calories or 66 pounds of potential body fat if this energy is not used as fuel for daily living.

High-carbohydrate diets that are especially high in sugar may be hazardous to one's health. They can increase the amount of triglycerides produced in the liver. These triglycerides are blood fats and are possible developers of hardened arteries. Also, a diet high in simple carbohydrates can lead to obesity, which can then result in the development of late-onset diabetes.

Fiber

Fiber is that part of the foods we take in that is not digestible. Fiber helps to move food through the intestines by increasing their peristaltic action. Vegetable fibers are made up chiefly of cellulose, an indigestible carbohydrate that is the main ingredient in the cell walls of plants. Plant-eating animals, such as cows, can digest cellulose. Meat-eating animals, such as humans, do not have the proper enzymes in their digestive tracts to metabolize cellulose.

Bran—the husks of wheat, oats, rice, rye, and corn—is another type of fiber. Bran is indigestible because of the silica in the outer husks. Some fibers, such as wheat bran, are also insoluble. The major function of fiber is to add bulk to the feces and to speed digested foods through the intestines. This reduces one's risk of constipation, intestinal cancer, appendicitis, and diverticulosis.

Some types of fibers are soluble; that is, they can find and eliminate certain substances such as dietary cholesterol. Pectin, commonly found in raw fruits (especially apple skins), oat and rice brans, and some gums from the seeds and stems of tropical plants (such as guar and xanthin) are examples of soluble fibers that pick up cholesterols as they move through the intestines.

Foods high in fiber are also valuable in weight-reducing diets because when foods pass more quickly through the digestive tract, the time available for absorption is reduced. Fiber also cuts the amount of hunger experienced by a dieter because it fills the stomach. A large salad with a diet dressing might give you very few calories, but it contains enough cellulose to fill your stomach, cut hunger, and move other foods through the intestinal passage.

Food processing often removes natural fiber from our food, and this is one of the primary reasons that we in the western world have relatively low amounts of fiber in our diet. For instance, white bread has only a trace of fiber—about nine grams in a loaf—while old-fashioned whole wheat bread has 70 grams. And when you peel a carrot or an apple, you remove much of the fiber.

Dietitians urge us to include more fiber in our diets. People should be particularly conscious of the benefits of whole-grain cereals, bran, and fibrous vegetables. Root vegetables (carrots, beets, and turnips) and leafy vegetables are very good sources of fiber. The average American diet has between 10 and 20 grams of fiber in it per day. This low level of fiber is believed to account for the

---

✓ *Checklist for Effective Eating*

1. Eat 12 to 15 percent of your diet in proteins, preferably fish, fowl without skin, and beans.
2. Keep your fat intake between 10 and 30 percent of your total calorie intake, with saturated fat intake 10 percent or less and a higher proportion of monounsaturated fat.
3. Most of your diet should be complex carbohydrates (less-refined products) such as whole wheat, fruits, and vegetables.
4. It is recommended that people supplement with antioxidant vitamins (beta carotene, vitamins C and E).

---

fact that we have about twice the rate of colon cancer as do other countries whose citizens eat more fiber. This is why the National Cancer Institute has recommended that we consume between 25 and 35 grams of fiber per day.

Vitamins

Vitamins are organic compounds that are essential in small amounts for the growth and development of animals and humans. They act as enzymes (catalysts) that facilitate many of the body's processes. Although there is controversy about the effects of consuming excess vitamins, nutritionists agree that we need a minimum amount of vitamins for proper functioning.

Some vitamins are soluble only in water; others need fat to be absorbed by the body. The water-soluble vitamins, B complex and C, are more fragile than the fat-soluble vitamins, because they are more easily destroyed by the heat of cooking, and if they are boiled, they lose some of their potency into the water. Since they are not stored by the body, they should be included in the daily diet. However, even though they are not stored in the body, it is still possible to ingest too many water-soluble vitamins, leading to kidney stones because of the excess demand placed on the kidneys for processing.

The fat-soluble vitamins, A, D, E, and K, need oils in the intestines to be absorbed by the body. They are more stable than the water-soluble vitamins and are not destroyed by normal cooking methods. Because they are stored in the body, there is the possibility of ingesting too much of them—especially vitamins A and D.

Although nutritional researchers disagree about whether vitamin supplements are necessary, many of them see the necessity for supplementation with the vitamins that neutralize free oxygen radicals. Free oxygen radicals are harmful substances produced by many natural body processes, air pollution, and smoke, and seem to be responsible for some cancers and other diseases. Physical exercise, for all of its benefits, is one producer of free oxygen radicals.

Supplementation with antioxidants (beta carotene, vitamins C and E) reduces free oxygen radicals in the body. Dr. Ken Cooper, the man who coined the term "aerobics" and developed the first world-recognized fitness program, suggests a minimum supplementation of 400 IU of vitamin E, 1,000 mg of vitamin C, and 25,000 of beta carotene daily to counteract the potential damage done to the body by free oxygen radicals.

Minerals

Minerals are usually structural components of the body, but they sometimes participate in certain body processes. The body uses many minerals: phosphorus, calcium, and magnesium for strong teeth and bones; zinc for growth; chromium for carbohydrate metabolism; and copper and iron for hemoglobin production in the blood.

Iron is used primarily in developing hemoglobin, which carries oxygen in red blood cells. Women need more iron (18 milligrams a day) than men until they go through menopause, at which time their iron requirements drop to that of men (10 milligrams a day). Iron deficiency, common in women athletes, may impair athletic performance and should be corrected with supplementation.

Magnesium is the eighth most abundant element on the earth's surface. It seems to help activate enzymes essential to energy transfer. It is crucial for effective contraction of the muscles. Exercise depletes this element, so supplementation may be called for. When it is not present in sufficient amounts, twitching, tremors, and undue anxiety may develop.

Calcium is primarily responsible for building strong bones and teeth. For this reason, it seems obvious that a diet that is chronically low in calcium would have a negative effect on one's bone strength. Low calcium intake results in brittle and porous bones as one gets older, a condition known as osteoporosis. This is diagnosed when bone density shows a loss of 40 percent of the necessary calcium. It happens quite often in older people, especially women who have gone through menopause or have had their ovaries removed, because estrogen seems to protect against bone loss.

In teenage and young adult years, the inclusion of adequate calcium (which may be higher than the current Recommended Daily Allowance, or RDA) can aid in the development of peak bone mass, which can help prevent osteoporosis later on in life. Another contributing factor to osteoporosis is the imbalance of phosphorus to calcium in the typical diet. Calcium and phosphorous work together, and should be consumed on a one-to-one ratio. However, the average diet is much higher in phosphorus than calcium, leading to a leaching of calcium from the bones to make up for this imbalance.

Calcium is also necessary for strong teeth, nerve transmissions, blood clotting, and muscle contractions. Without enough calcium, muscle cramps often result. Skipping milk with its necessary calcium may be the cause of menstrual cramping for some girls. The uterus is a muscle, and muscles need both sodium and calcium for proper contractile functioning.

Phytochemicals

Phytochemicals (phyto is the Greek word for "plant") include thousands of chemical compounds that are found in plants. Some of these are vitamins and many have no known effect on us; however, more and more are being found to be highly beneficial.

In the past, the phytonutrients found in fruits and vegetables were classified as vitamins: Flavonoids were known as vitamin P, cabbage factors (glucosinolates and indoles) were called vitamin U, and ubiquinone was vitamin Q. Tocopherol somehow stayed on the list as vitamin E. The vitamin designation was dropped for other nutrients because specific deficiency symptoms could not be established. "Vita" means "life," so if the compound could not be found to be absolutely essential for life, it was dropped as a "vitamin," but is now classified as a phytochemical.

Various phytochemicals have been found to reduce the chance of cancers developing, reduce the chance of heart attack, reduce blood pressure, and increase immunity factors. Few of these have been reduced to pill form, such as vitamin pills, so they must be consumed in fruits and vegetables daily. It is suggested that each of us consume at least five servings of raw fruits or vegetables daily. Since many of the phytochemicals are heat sensitive, cooking can destroy some or all of the active ingredients.

We are a long way from developing highly effective phytochemical supplements, because there are so many elements and they may be destroyed in the processing. Garlic pills, for example, are available. However, in the deodorized versions, some active ingredients have been removed—they were in the chemicals that give garlic its "aroma."

Several types of phytochemicals are being studied. *Plant sterols* are somewhat similar to the animal sterol cholesterol but are unsaturated. These plant sterols compete for the same sites and thereby lower the blood cholesterol levels by as much as 10 percent. Soy is a good source for such sterols. Most green and yellow vegetables, and particularly their seeds, contain essential sterols.

Phenols have the ability to block specific enzymes that cause inflammation. They also modify the prostaglandin pathways and thereby protect blood platelets from clumping, thereby reducing the risk of blood clots. Blue, blue-red, and violet colorations seen in berries, grapes, and purple eggplant are due to their phenolic content.

Flavonoids is the name for a large group of compounds found primarily in tea, citrus fruits, onions, soy, and wine. Some can be irritating, but others seem to reduce heart attack risk. For example, the phenolic substances in red wine inhibit oxidation of human LDL cholesterol. The biologic activities of flavonoids include action against allergies, inflammation, free radicals, liver toxins, blood clotting, ulcers, viruses, and tumors.

Terpenes such as those found in green foods, soy products, and grains comprise one of the largest classes of phytonutrients. The most intensely studied terpenes are carotenoids—as evidenced by the many recent studies on beta carotene. Only a few of the carotenoids have the antioxidant properties of beta carotene. These substances are found in bright yellow, orange, and red plant pigments found in vegetables such as tomatoes, parsley, oranges, pink grapefruit, and spinach.

Limonoids are a subclass of terpenes found in citrus fruit peels. They appear to protect lung tissue and aid in detoxifying harmful chemicals in the liver.

Recent research confirms suspicion of the effects of soy products and related foods, which have long been used in Oriental diets. It has long been observed that Oriental women do not experience the problems of menopause, such as hot flashes, that western women commonly endure, but until recently, no theories have been advanced. Now we realize that a major factor is the fact that the Asians eat more vegetables, particularly soybeans.

It is phytoestrogens—plant chemicals that mimic the effects of the female hormone estrogen—that seem to be the major factor. These plant-like estrogens have similar effects to the natural estrogen in reducing heart disease, maintaining brain functions, reducing the incidence of breast cancer, and reducing softening of the bones (osteoporosis). In addition, other positive effects, which may or may not be related to estrogen intake, also occur, such as reduction in cancers (prostate, endometrial, bowel) and the effects of alcohol abuse[1].

Water

Water is called the essential nonnutrient because it has no nutritional value, yet without it we would die. Water makes up approximately 60 percent of the adult body, while an infant's body is nearly 80 percent water. Water cools the body through perspiration, carries nutrients to and waste products from the cells, helps cushion our vital organs, and is an essential element of all body fluids.

The body has about 18 square feet of skin that contains about 2 million sweat glands. On a comfortable day, a person perspires about a half-pint of water. Somebody exercising on a severely hot day may lose as much as seven quarts of water. If this is not replaced, severe dehydration can result. It is therefore generally recommended that we daily drink eight 8-ounce glasses of water or the equivalent in other fluids. This amount is dependent on the climate in which you live, the altitude at which you live, the type of foods that you eat, and the amount of activity that you participate in on a day-to-day basis. Tennis can be very strenuous and makes us sweat—so be sure to drink plenty of water during practice or games. Chapter 17 discusses fluid replacement in greater detail.

---

[1] S. A. Bingham et al., "Phyto-oestrogens: Where are we now?" *British Journal of Nutrition*, May 1998, 79(5) 393–406; S. T. Willard and L. S. Frawley, ""Phytoestrogens have agonistic and combinatorial effects on estrogen-responsive gene expression in MCF-7 human breast cancer cells," *Endocrinology*, April 1998, 8(2), 117–121; T. B. Clarkson, "The potential of soybean phytoestrogens for postmenopausal hormone replacement therapy," *Proceedings of the Society of Experimental Biological Medicine*, March 1998, 217(3), 365–368.

Summary

1. The basic macronutrients are proteins, fats, and carbohydrates.
2. Proteins are made of amino acids. Eight of these are considered to be essential and should be consumed daily.
3. Our bodies need fats, but they should be limited to 10 to 20 percent of our daily calorie intake.
4. Saturated fats and cholesterol are risk factors for heart disease.
5. The greatest percentage of our diets should be in complex carbohydrates, which contain vitamins, minerals, and fiber.
6. While proteins, fats, and carbohydrates (macronutrients) provide most of the nutrients we consume, the micronutrients (vitamins, minerals, and phytochemicals) are also essential.
7. Vitamins break down macronutrients and accomplish other essential body functions.
8. Free oxygen radicals are harmful byproducts of living that can be reduced by some vitamins (beta carotene, vitamins C and E).
9. Minerals are necessary building blocks of the body and are essential in all tissue.
10. Phytochemicals are desirable—and possibly necessary—elements found in plants, and may aid us in obtaining a higher level of nutrition.
11. Vitamin supplementation may be necessary for many people; most of us apparently profit from antioxidant supplementation.
12. Water is essential to all the body's functions; eight glasses of water a day is recommended.

16 Sensible Eating and Weight Management

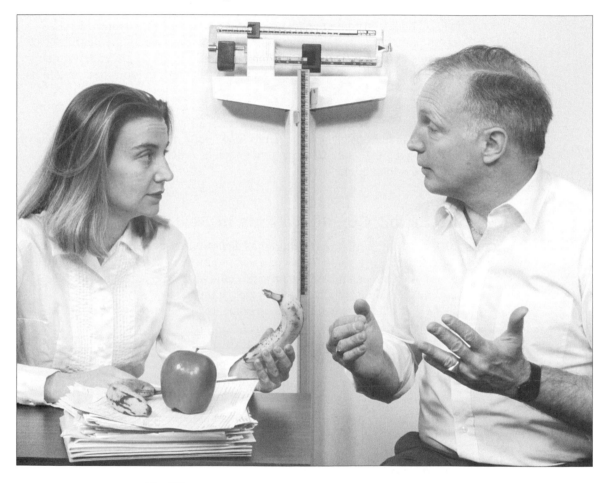

Outline

To eat sensibly, you must understand the basic principles of nutrition discussed in Chapter 15. Necessary nutrients must occur in your diet in proper quantities, and the calories you consume must be the amount necessary in order to maintain your desired weight. If you don't maintain your optimal weight, you may develop obesity and the diseases associated with obesity, such as diabetes, high blood pressure, and heart disease.

There are other factors that the sensible eater must understand. Caloric needs change according to climate and the amount of activity in which the person participates. For example, hot weather necessitates a greater intake of fluids due to the loss of water through perspiration, and you need fewer calories because your body does not need to burn as many calories to maintain its 98.6° Fahrenheit temperature.

A person using a great many calories, such as a tennis player, needs more carbohydrates, but it is a myth that athletes need a great deal more protein than non-athletes. While caloric needs may nearly double for the athlete who is expending a great deal of energy, protein needs are increased only slightly—usually less than 30 percent.

Important Considerations in Selecting Your Diet

The U.S. Department of Agriculture has devised a suggested diet guide called the Food Guide Pyramid. Its base is grain products, next comes fruits and vegetables, then meats and animal products, and at the top some fats or sweets if needed. There are six food groups in the pyramid:

- Grain products (breads, cereals, pastas): six to eleven servings per day recommended
- Vegetables: three to five servings per day recommended
- Fruits: two to four servings per day recommended
- High-protein meats and meat substitutes (meat, poultry, fish, beans, nuts, tofu/soy, eggs): two to three servings per day recommended
- Milk products: two servings per day for adults, three for children recommended
- Extra calories, if needed, from fats and/or sweets

Grain products provide the carbohydrates needed for quick energy. A serving size is one slice of bread, an ounce of dry cereal, or a half-cup of cooked cereal, pasta, or rice. Daily needs are six to eleven servings.

Grains are rich in B vitamins, some minerals, and fiber. Whole grains are the best sources of fibers. Refining grains or polishing rice reduces the fiber, the mineral content, and the B vitamins. This occurs in white and wheat bread (not whole wheat), pastas, pastries, and white rice. Flour is often refortified with three of the B complex vitamins, but seldom with the other essential nutrients.

If you want to reduce your cholesterol level, thereby reducing your chances of heart disease, reduce your chances of developing gallstones, or have a softer bowel movement, eat more of the soluble fibers (oat bran cereals, whole grain

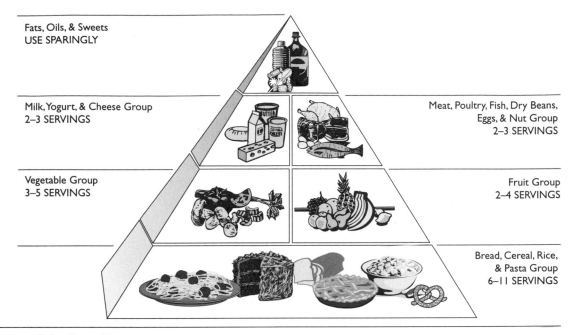

Fats, Oils, & Sweets
USE SPARINGLY

Milk, Yogurt, & Cheese Group
2–3 SERVINGS

Meat, Poultry, Fish, Dry Beans,
Eggs, & Nut Group
2–3 SERVINGS

Vegetable Group
3–5 SERVINGS

Fruit Group
2–4 SERVINGS

Bread, Cereal, Rice,
& Pasta Group
6–11 SERVINGS

The Food Guide Pyramid

bread with oats, rice bran, carrots, potatoes, apples, and citrus juices that contain pulp). If your concern is reducing your risk of intestinal cancers, appendicitis, and diverticulosis, eat more of the insoluble fibers (whole wheat breads and cereals, corn cereals, prunes, beans, peas, nuts, most vegetables, and polished rice).

Vegetables are rich in fibers, beta carotene, some vitamins, and minerals. Among the most nutritious vegetables are broccoli, carrots, peas, peppers, and sweet potatoes. If you are trying to lose weight, many vegetables are high in water and in fibers but low in calories. Among these are all greens (lettuce, cabbage, celery) as well as cauliflower. Actually, most vegetables are quite low in calories. You need three to five servings daily; a serving size is a half-cup of raw or cooked vegetables or a cup of raw leafy vegetables.

Fruits are generally high in vitamin C and fiber, and they are also relatively low in calories. You should have two to four servings daily; a serving size is one-fourth cup of dried fruit, a half-cup of cooked fruit, three-quarters cup of fruit juice, a whole piece of fruit, or a wedge of a melon.

Protein sources such as meats, egg whites, nuts, and beans are also high in minerals and vitamins B-6 and B-12. You need two to three servings a day; a serving is two and one-half ounces of cooked meat, poultry or fish, two egg whites, four tablespoons of peanut butter, one and one-fourth cups of cooked beans. A McDonald's "Quarter-Pounder" would give you two servings. The hidden eggs in cakes and cookies also count. The best meat products to eat are fish, egg whites, and poultry without the skin.

Red meat not only has a relatively low quality of protein (ranked after egg white, milk, fish, poultry, and organ meats), but it is linked to both cancers (two and a half times the risk for colon cancer) and heart disease. It also carries a great amount of fat, even if the fat on the outside is trimmed off. There is also a lot of cholesterol in the meat and fat of all land animals. Taking the skin off poultry greatly reduces the amount of fat and cholesterol that will be consumed, because poultry carry much of their fat next to the skin.

Of the animal proteins, fish has a higher quality of protein than meat or poultry. Also, fish are able to convert polyunsaturated linolenic fatty acids from plants they eat into omega 3 oils, which work to prevent heart disease by reducing cholesterol and by making the blood less likely to clot in the arteries. They do this by interfering with the body's production of the prostaglandin thromboxane, which increases blood clotting.

Milk and milk products (cheeses, yogurt, ice cream) are high in calcium and protein as well as in some minerals (potassium and zinc) and riboflavin. Adults need two servings daily, while children need three; a serving is one cup of milk or yogurt, one and one-half ounces of cheese, two cups of cottage cheese, one and one-half cups of ice cream, or one cup of pudding or custard.

Fats and sweets are positioned at the top of the pyramid of foods. They should be eaten only if a person needs extra calories. Consuming more fat than the recommended maximum of 30 percent of one's diet can be quite harmful—particularly in causing cancers and hardened arteries. Most researchers suggest a maximum of 10 to 20 percent of the diet in fats, with most in the form of monounsaturated and polyunsaturated fatty acids.

Sweets may assist in the development of tooth caries (cavities), but are not otherwise harmful if calories are not a problem for you. An athlete consuming 5,000 calories in a day can probably eat candy bars and ice cream, but the person attempting to control their weight should avoid them.

In addition to merely consuming the right proportions of foods, a concerned person would implement several other precautions:

- Avoid milk fat by drinking nonfat milk and milk products; eating ice milk (3 percent fat) or frozen desserts made without milk fat; and eating no-fat or low-fat cheeses. Half of the calories in whole milk come from the 3 ½ percent of the milk that is fat. Low-fat milk is reduced in fat calories by 40 percent. When low-fat milk is advertised as 98 percent fat-free, it is not that much better than whole milk, which is 96 ½ percent fat-free. The fats in milk are highly saturated—the worst kind of fat—yet the protein quality of milk is second only to egg whites.

- Avoid egg yolks because they contain a great deal of cholesterol and saturated fat. They are second only to caviar (fish eggs) in cholesterol content. Egg whites, on the other hand, have the highest rating for protein quality and are one of the best things you can eat.

- Reduce salt, because it is related to high blood pressure; and sugars, because they give "empty" calories—calories without other nutrients such as vitamins or fiber.

- Reduce fats to between 10 and 20 percent of your total calories. Normal salad dressings contain about 70 calories per tablespoon. If calories are a problem, use fat-free dressing or vinegar or lemon juice only. Rather than a butter or margarine, buy a good tasty whole-grain bread and eat it without grease. If you must use grease, use olive oil, or perhaps olive oil and balsamic vinegar as they serve in many Italian restaurants. If calories are not a concern and you like sweets, use jelly or jam.

- Never fry foods in oil; use a non-stick pan. If you must have an oil, use canola (rapeseed), olive, or safflower oil. Stay away from all fried foods, including potato chips. Fried foods not only add calories and saturated fats, but they also increase one's chances for intestinal cancers—as do all fats.

Beverages

Beverages make up a large part of our diet. We often don't think too much about the kinds of liquids we drink. The most nutritious drinks have been rated by the Center for Science in the Public Interest according to the amount of fat and sugar (higher content = lower rating), and their amount of protein, vitamins, and minerals (higher content = higher rating). Here are some sample results: skim or nonfat milk was rated +47, whole milk +38 (the lower rating was because of its fat content), orange juice +33, Hi-C +4, coffee 0, coffee with cream –1, coffee with sugar –12, Kool-Aid –55, and soft drinks –92.

Milk is the best beverage for most people. Children should have three to four cups each day, while adults should drink two cups. Our need for milk can be satisfied by other dairy products. For example, two cups of milk are equivalent to three cups of cottage cheese or five large scoops of ice cream. (Of course, this choice may *taste* the best, but there are obvious drawbacks to eating five scoops of ice cream every day!) In addition to its nutritional value as a developer of bones and organs, milk has been found to help people sleep. People who drink milk at night go to sleep more quickly, and sleep longer and sounder. This is because of the high content of the amino acid tryptophan, which makes serotonin, the neurotransmitter (brain chemical) associated with relaxation and calming.

Coffee contains several ingredients that may be harmful to the body. There are stimulants such as caffeine and the xanthines, as well as oils that seem to stimulate the secretion of excess acid in the stomach. And there are diuretics that eliminate water and some nutrients, such as calcium, from the body. Even two cups a day increases the risk of bone fractures[1]. A factor that may add to the risk of bone fractures is that people who drink more coffee usually drink little or no milk.

---

[1] E. Barrett-Connor, "Caffeine and bone fractures," *Journal of the American Medical Association*, January 26, 1994.

Caffeine is found in coffee, tea, and cola and many other drinks. Brewed coffee contains 100 to 150 milligrams of caffeine per cup (mg/cup), instant coffee about 90 mg/cup, tea between 45 and 75 mg/cup, and cola drinks from 40 to 60 mg/cup. Decaffeinated coffee is virtually free of caffeine, containing only two to four mg/cup. The therapeutic dose of caffeine given to people who have overdosed on barbiturates is 43 milligrams. Yet a cup of coffee contains up to 150 milligrams of caffeine!

Caffeine is a central nervous system stimulant. It elevates your blood pressure and constricts your blood vessels, both of which effects may assist in the development of high blood pressure. It has also been reported that excess caffeine in coffee, tea, and cola drinks can produce the same symptoms found in someone suffering from psychological anxiety, including nervousness, irritability, occasional muscle twitching, sensory disturbances, diarrhea, insomnia, irregular heartbeat, a drop in blood pressure, and occasionally failures of the blood circulation system.

Coffee is an irritant. The oils in coffee irritate the lining of the stomach and the upper intestines. People who drink two or more cups of coffee per day increase their chances of getting ulcers by 72 percent over non–coffee drinkers. Decaffeinated coffee is no more soothing to the ulcer patient than the regular blend, because both types increase the acid secretions in the stomach. Since an ulcer patient's acid secretion is not as high when caffeine alone is ingested (when compared to the acid levels after the ingestion of decaffeinated coffee), some other ingredient in coffee is thought to be responsible for these increased stomach acid levels.

Tea is not as irritating as coffee, but it does contain some caffeine and tannic acid, which can irritate the stomach. If you drink large amounts of tea, you should either take it with milk to neutralize the acid or add ice to dilute it. Green tea, the type commonly drunk in Asia, contains polyphenols, which appear to be antioxidants and may reduce cancer incidence. Black tea, the kind commonly drunk in Europe and America, has less of these protective substances[2]. Not much is known about the effects of herbal teas.

Alcohol contains seven calories per gram. These calories contain no nutritional elements, but they do contribute to your total caloric intake. Since alcoholic drinks are surprisingly high in calories, they contribute to the overweight problems of many individuals. People who drink alcoholic beverages and eat a balanced diet will probably consume too many calories. If they drink but cut down on eating, they may not develop a weight problem, but they will probably develop nutritional deficiencies that can result in severe illness. Alcohol is also a central nervous system depressant, which causes a decrease in one's metabolism.

---

[2] *University of California, Berkeley Wellness Letter*, January 1992, pp. 1–2.

In addition to the normal dangers of alcohol in creating alcoholism and destroying brain cells, there are other considerations in drinking. Beer or ale, because of their carbonation, have the effect of neutralizing stomach acid. This can increase the acids secreted by the stomach, causing ulcers.

Food Additives

Sugar is a negative for most people. In fact it is probably the most harmful additive to the foods that we in the United States eat. We average about 125 pounds of sugar per person per year. This gives us a lot of excess calories that, if not used for energy, will be stored as fat. As discussed previously, if we exceed our desired weight and become obese, we will have increased health risks.

Salt can be a dangerous food additive, yet most people do not consider adding salt to their food to be a health risk. But when you look at populations as a whole, it seems obvious that the higher the salt intake, the greater the frequency of high blood pressure.

Many manufacturers add salt to enhance the taste of food, and sodium is often high in processed or canned foods. While the desired intake is between one and two grams (1,000 and 2,000 milligrams), the average daily intake in America is five grams. The potential negative effect of a high sodium intake can be combated by ingesting a high level of potassium. However, the desired recommended daily allowance for potassium, 2.5 grams, is not met by the average American, who consumes only 0.8 to 1.5 grams daily. Most of our foods follow this same pattern—too high in sodium and too low in potassium.

Preservatives added to foods lengthen storage life and prevent disease-causing germs from multiplying. Most are harmless, and some give protection against intestinal cancers. Some, however, such as the nitrates in hot dogs, have been implicated in causing cancer. Nevertheless, the disease of botulism, which they prevent, is far more of a danger than that posed by the nitrates.

Vitamins and minerals have been added to food for years. In 1973, the Food and Drug Administration suggested that more iron be added to enrich flour after they found that iron is often low in our diets. Vitamins A and D are added to skim milk to make it nonfat milk—milk that has all of the nutrients of whole milk but without the fat. Vitamins A and D are fat soluble and stay in the fat when it is removed to make skim milk.

Vegetarianism

When vegetarians are careful about their dietary intakes, they may prove to be healthier than nonvegetarians. One study comparing healthy vegetarians to nonvegetarians found that healthy vegetarians had lower blood sugar and cholesterol levels than did their closely matched nonvegetarian counterparts.

Smart Shopping

Shopping for low-fat foods requires a sharp eye. If you are looking for a low-fat food, look at the total grams of fat, multiply by nine (nine calories per gram of fat), then divide that by the total number of calories in the food. (For example, if a food has three grams of fat, nine times that equals 27 total calories from fat. If the food has a total of 270 calories, then the percentage of fat calories is 10 percent.) If the food has one of the new food labels, it will list both the number of fat values and the approximate percentage of fat calories per serving. You want to keep your daily total percentage of fat below 30 percent to decrease your risk of developing heart disease. Even better than the suggested maximum of 30 percent is keeping the total to 10 or 20 percent fat.

Many foods, particularly low-fat liquids such as salad dressings without oil, have replaced the oil with some gums. Guar, locust bean, and xanthine gums are soluble fibers that help remove cholesterol from the intestines. So you get a double advantage—no fat and some cholesterol-removal substances.

The food label lists ingredients according to their content in the product. The higher on the list of ingredients, the more of that item is present in the food. So if the product lists wheat flour first, there is no problem. But if it lists eggs or hydrogenated oils second, the food may be too high in fat. And if you are watching your sodium intake, remember to look for salt on the list.

Eating and Overeating

People eat to nourish their bodies. But in America many people eat to reduce stress. We may not be satisfied in our work, at school, or in our relationships, but we can be satiated with food. Filling our stomachs can make us feel that in at least one part of our lives we are totally satisfied. When we eat to relieve stress, we will probably take in more calories than we need for living—but even worse, stress eating often means junk foods. It is much more intelligent to play some tennis to relieve stress.

Being overweight is a more common concern than is being underweight. While some people are overweight, some are obese. For example, 35 percent of women are 20 percent overweight.[3] Of people who are obese, one in 20 has a genetic factor or a problem in physical malfunctioning, such as an underactive thyroid, a problem with the hypothalamus, or one of the other centers of the brain that deals with whether or not we feel full or hungry. There are medical procedures that can help these people. In cases where the metabolism is slowed, such as by an underactive thyroid gland, doctors can administer the proper hormone to increase metabolism back into what is considered a normal range.

---

[3] *Harvard Women's Health Watch*, November 1994, p. 4.

Another cause of obesity is thought to be the number of fat cells in a person's body. This is known as the *set point theory*. It is thought that the more fat cells one has, the more one is driven to eat to maintain these fat cells. The number of fat cells one has is generally set after puberty.

For others, obesity is caused by overeating to an extreme degree. However, according to the Harvard University Nutrition Department, most people are overfat because they don't exercise, not because they overeat. Overeating coupled with a lack of exercise is a sure way to become obese.

Since it is the amount of body fat that a person carries that is the true culprit of disease, it is preferable to refer to this health risk as being overfat rather than being overweight. Many bodybuilders may be overweight when compared to the height/weight charts commonly used to measure health risks by insurance companies, but they are not overfat.

Determining if you are overfat can be done in several ways. The most common method is to look at yourself in a mirror. If you look fat, you may be fat. Another way is to pinch the fat you carry just below the skin. If you can pinch an inch, you are probably carrying too much fat. Professionals often use skin calipers to measure the amount of fat people carry in four to seven designated spots on the body, or they use underwater weighing or bioelectrical impedence.

Once your body fat percentage is determined, you can then find out what a healthy weight would be for you. Men are usually considered healthy if their body fat is in the range of 10 to 15 percent, while women are healthy if they fall between 18 to 25 percent body fat. Men are considered overfat if their body fat is over 20 percent, while women are overfat if their body fat is over 30 percent. Women require more fat than men do because of their menstrual cycle. If a woman falls below 12 percent body fat, she may become amenorrheic (lose her regular menstrual cycle).

Should You Lose Weight?

Before you decide to lose weight, you first need to determine whether your are overweight due to being overfat. From a health point of view, it is your proportion of fat and lean body mass that is most important.

How to Lose Weight

The wisest approach to losing weight would be to find out why you are overweight. If it is genetic, perhaps medical help is needed. If you eat because of stress, you should find another way to relieve stress, such as exercise or relaxation techniques or, if you must have something in your mouth, try gum or a low-calorie food. If your problem is a lack of exercise, start an effective exercise program. If you consume too many calories, you will need to change your diet.

Don't even start a weight-loss program if you are not willing to make lifestyle changes for the rest of your life. The great majority of dieters refuse to make such a commitment. That is why 40 percent of women and 25 percent of men are on a diet at any one time and the average American goes on 2.3 diets a year, and it is also why 95 percent of dieters regain all of their lost weight within five years. The average diet is just not successful.

In all likelihood, if you adopt the habits of effective exercise and a low-fat and low-alcohol eating pattern, the pounds will drop off. Losing weight just for the sake of being thinner seldom works for very long. You have to determine whether you honestly want a healthier lifestyle or just to look better for the summer. A pattern of continually gaining and losing weight is frustrating and probably not worth the effort. But a true lifestyle change to healthy eating and regular exercise will pay many mental, physical, and social dividends.

We must recognize that the fat we wear comes primarily from the fat we eat. Because carbohydrates are so efficiently converted to sugar glucose, they are used first for energy in the body. To convert carbohydrates to fat, about 23 percent of the energy is used to make the conversion. Protein, if not used, will normally be converted into sugars and will be the second source of available energy. But the fat you eat uses only 3 percent of its food value in the conversion to body fat.

So 25 grams of carbohydrate, which will yield 100 calories (at 4 calories a gram), is reduced by 23 percent of the calories used to convert them to body fat. But fats consumed in your food are different. Eleven grams of fat (at nine calories per gram) is 99 calories, but it only takes 3 percent of those calories to convert it all to body fat, and 96 calories of body fat can be deposited. So 100 calories of carbohydrates, if not used for energy, will become about 8.5 grams of body fat, but 100 calories of fat from the diet will become about 10.75 grams of body fat.

To lose one pound of fat per week, you must have a net deficit of 500 calories per day; one pound of fat contains 3,500 calories. You may choose to achieve this solely by decreasing your food intake by 500 calories per day.

You could also choose to increase your activity level to burn off 500 calories a day. Keep in mind that it takes a great deal of energy to achieve this goal, and it can be dangerous for you to embark on such a strenuous exercise program if you are not currently exercising. It is best to combine calorie reduction with exercise to achieve your goal. Aerobic exercise will keep your metabolism up as you lose the fat, and you won't have to restrict your calories as much because you will be burning off energy each time you exercise.

Playing singles tennis burns about 3.4 calories per pound per hour. For a 150-pound person, this is about 510 calories per hour.

We now know that calories are used both during and after exercise. The longer and more vigorous the exercise, the longer one's metabolism is increased, so that for more hours after the exercise is completed, the calorie expenditure will be increased over normal. While this increase in calories burned after one has finished exercising is not a large amount, it is still an increase over one's resting metabolism, and a calorie burned is a calorie burned!

Calories Burned with Various Activities

	Calories per pound per hour	Calories expended by 150 lb. person in 20 minutes
Sleeping	0.36	18.0
Sitting at rest	0.55	27.5
Sitting at work	0.60	30.0
Light exercise (housework)	1.00	50.0
Walking	1.20	60.0
Jogging (slow)	1.75	87.5
Volleyball (recreational 6-person)	1.50	65.0
Tennis	3.40	154

Some people think that exercising will make them eat more. A quarter-mile to a mile of jogging or a good set of tennis games will have no measurable effect on the total intake of calories. In fact, by exercising just before a meal, you can dull your appetite and decrease your desire for more calories.

Eating Disorders

Anorexia nervosa is starvation by choice. This is a disease primarily seen in young women. It afflicts nearly one in a hundred women, although 5 to 10 percent of its victims are male. In this disease, the person goes on a diet and refuses to stop, no matter how thin he or she gets. About one out of ten people who have this disorder end up starving themselves to death. The disease has a psychological basis, but its physical effects are very real. Medical care, usually hospitalization, is generally required.

After the anorexic begins the severe dieting routine, symptoms of starvation may set in, leading to a number of physical problems. Abnormal thyroid, adrenal, and growth hormone functions are not uncommon. The heart muscle becomes weakened. Amenorrhea occurs in women and girls due to the low percentage of body fat. Blood pressure may drop. Anemia is common due to the lack of protein and iron ingested. The peristalsis of the intestines may slow and the lining of the intestines may atrophy. The pancreas often becomes unable to secrete many of its enzymes. Body temperature may drop. The skin may become dry and there can be an increase of body hair in the body's attempt to keep itself warm. And for 10 percent of sufferers, the result is death.

Because dieting is such a common occurrence in our society, anorexia is often difficult to diagnose until the person has entered the advanced stages of the disease. However, other symptoms such as moodiness, being withdrawn, obsessing about food but never being seen eating it, and constant food preparation may be observed by those close to the anorexic. Once diagnosed, there are a number of medical and psychological therapies that can be effective.

Bulimia, or *bulimia nervosa*, is more common than anorexia. The person with bulimia restricts calorie intake during the day, but binges on high-fat, high-calorie foods at least twice a week. Following the binge, the person purges in an attempt to get rid of the excess calories just consumed. Purging techniques include vomiting, laxatives, fasting, and excessive exercise. Some experts do not consider the behavior bulimic until it has persisted for about three months with two or more binges per week during that time. Estimates based on various surveys of college students and others indicate that between 5 and 20 percent of women may be bulimic. It is also more common among men than is anorexia.

Bulimia, like anorexia, stems from a psychological problem. However, in some cases there may also be a link to physical abnormalities. The neurotransmitters serotonin and norepinephrine seem to be involved, as does the hormone cholecystokinin, which is secreted by the hypothalamus and makes a person feel that enough food has been eaten.

Physical symptoms to look for depend on the type of purging technique used. The bulimic who induces vomiting can have scars on the back of the knuckles, mouth sores, gingivitis, tooth decay, a swollen esophagus, and chronic bad breath. The bulimic who uses laxatives has constant diarrhea, which can cause irreparable damage to the intestines. All bulimics run the risk of throwing off their electrolytes (minerals involved in muscle contractions) as a result of constant dehydration. It is this imbalance of electrolytes that can cause the bulimic to have abnormal heart rhythms and that can induce a heart attack.

Female athletes sometimes develop problems called the "female athletic triad,"[4] or a combination of eating disorders, osteoporosis, and amenorrhea. It is caused by the hard training practiced by competitive athletes or dancers and the desire to keep weight low, which often results in inadequate nutrition. Weight loss is sometimes achieved by bulimic methods. The result is weight that is too low, a loss of calcium from the bones, and a lack of healthy menstruation.

These problems are most likely to occur in activities in which low weight is an advantage, such as dancing, distance running, figure skating, and gymnastics, and it is more prevalent among athletes in individual sports than in team sports. Males, with the exception of competitive wrestlers, do not often experience the need to eat less. While this disorder doesn't generally affect tennis players, you should be aware of the problem.

---

[4] Aurelia Nattiv, Barbara Drinkwater, et al. "The female athletic triad," *Clinics in Sports Medicine: The Athletic Woman*, W. B. Saunders: Philadelphia, 13(2), April 1994, pp. 405–418.

Summary

1. Sensible eating requires some understanding of the science of nutrition.
2. Following the guidelines of the Food Pyramid will generally give a person an adequate diet.
3. Skim or nonfat milk is the best beverage.
4. Salt and sugar are the most common food additives.
5. Many people overeat and become overfat.
6. Most overfat people can lose weight through an effective diet and adequate exercise.
7. Eating disorders seem to be prevalent; anorexia nervosa and bulimia are the major eating disorders.

Self-Test

Write in the number that best describes your eating habits:

3—Almost always   2—Sometimes   1—Almost never

____ 1. Do you eat three or more pieces of fruit per day? (Fruit juice counts as one piece.)
____ 2. Do you eat a minimum of three servings of vegetables each day—including a green leafy or orange vegetable?
____ 3. Do you eat three or four milk products (such as milk, cheese, yogurt) per day?
____ 4. Do you eat a minimum of six servings of grain products (breads, cereal, pasta) each day?
____ 5. Do you eat breakfast?
____ 6. Do you eat fish at least three times per week?
____ 7. Do you avoid fried foods, including potato chips and french fries?
____ 8. Do you eat fast food fewer than three times per week?
____ 9. Are the milk products you consume made from nonfat milk?
____ 10. Do you avoid high-sugar foods and highly refined carbohydrates such as sweet rolls, cookies, nondiet sodas, candy, etc.?

Your Score

25–30   You are balancing your diet well.
18–24   Your diet needs to be improved.
10–17   Your diet is unhealthy.

Bulimia Self-Test

Write "Never," "Sometimes," or "Often" to describe your weight-control practices:

____ 1. Is your life a series of constant diets?
____ 2. Do you vomit or take laxatives or diuretics to control your weight?
____ 3. Do you alternate periods of eating binges with fasts to control your weight?
____ 4. Does your weight fluctuate by as much as 10 pounds because of eating habits?
____ 5. Have you ever had a "food binge" during which you ate a large amount of food in a short period of time?
____ 6. If you "binged," was it on high-calorie food such as ice cream, cookies, donuts, or cake?
____ 7. Have you ever stopped a binge by vomiting, sleeping, or experiencing pain?
____ 8. Do you think your eating habits vary from the average person's?
____ 9. Are you out of control with your eating habits?
____10. Are you close to 100 pounds overweight because of your eating habits?

If you marked two or more of the above questions "Often," you may have a serious eating disorder called *bulimia*.

Where to Go for Help

Anorexia Bulimia Treatment Education Center: 800-33-ABTEC
Bulimia Anorexia Self-Help: 800-227-4785
Low-fat diet gourmet meals are possible. Send for the free *Metropolitan Cookbook*. Write to: Health and Welfare Department, Metropolitan Life Insurance Co., 1 Madison Avenue, New York, NY 10010) . Or buy the American Heart Association's cookbook.

Height and Weight Table: Men*

Height	Small Frame	Medium Frame	Large Frame
5'2"	128–134	131–141	138–150
5'3"	130–136	133–143	140–153
5'4"	132–138	135–145	142–156
5'5"	134–140	137–148	144–160
5'6"	136–142	139–151	146–164
5'7"	138–145	142–154	149–168
5'8"	140–148	145–157	152–172
5'9"	142–151	148–160	155–176
5'10"	144–154	151–163	158–180
5'11"	146–157	154–166	161–184
6'0"	149–160	157–170	164–188
6'1"	152–164	160–174	168–192
6'2"	155–168	164–178	172–197
6'3"	158–172	167–182	176–202
6'4"	162–176	171–187	181–207

*Weights at ages 25 to 59 based on lowest mortality. Weight in pounds according to frame (in indoor clothing weighing 5 lbs.; shoes with 1" heels).
Source: 1999 Metropolitan Life Insurance Company height and weight tables.

Height and Weight Table: Women†

Height	Small Frame	Medium Frame	Large Frame
4'10"	102–111	109–121	118–131
4'11"	103–113	111–123	120–134
5'0"	104–115	113–126	122–137
5'1"	106–118	115–129	125–140
5'2"	108–121	118–132	128–143
5'3"	111–124	121–135	131–147
5'4"	114–127	124–138	134–151
5'5"	117–130	127–141	137–155
5'6"	120–133	130–144	140–159
5'7"	123–136	133–147	143–163
5'8"	126–139	136–150	146–167
5'9"	129–142	139–153	149–170
5'10"	132–145	142–156	152–173
5'11"	135–148	145–159	155–176
6'0"	138–151	148–162	158–179

†Weights at ages 25 to 59 based on lowest mortality. Weight in pounds according to frame (in indoor clothing weighing 3 lbs.; shoes with 1" heels).
Source: 1999 Metropolitan Life Insurance Company height and weight tables.

17 Fluid Replacement and Problems of Heat and Cold

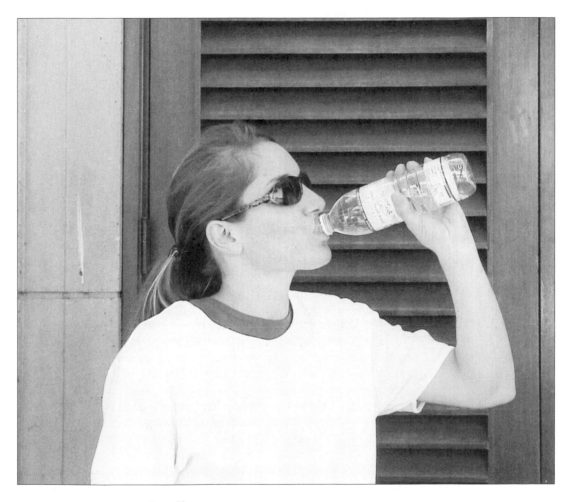

Outline

Heat
Cold
Problems Caused by Heat
Checklist for Preventing Heat-Related Problems
Summary

T ennis is often played in warm weather, and the activity can make you perspire. Therefore, when you play tennis, you should be aware of over-heating and proper rehydration.

Heat

Excess heat not only negatively affects your performance, but it also can be a source of serious health problems. As the outside temperature increases, it becomes more and more difficult for the body to rid itself of the heat that exercise produces. For example, if you are exercising at 37° F (3° C) you are 20 percent more effective in eliminating body heat than if you were exercising at 67° F (20° C) and 150 percent more effective than if you were exercising at 104° F (40° C). It is not uncommon for the body to reach a temperature of 104° to 106° F (40° to 41° C) when exercising. But normal resting body temperature is 98.6° F (37° C). The high heat makes it difficult, or impossible, for the perspiration to evaporate, and as a result, the body can't be effectively cooled.

The heat generated in the muscles is released by:

- Conduction—from the warmer muscles to the cooler skin
- Convection—from the the skin to the air
- Evaporation—of perspiration

Conduction occurs through the body's liquids, such as the blood, absorbing the heat created by the contraction of the muscles and moving it to the cooler skin. Water can absorb many thousands of times more heat than can air, so it is an excellent conductor of heat from the muscles.

Convection occurs when the heat near the skin is absorbed into the atmosphere. For a swimmer in a cool pool, effective convection is very easy. For the runner it is more difficult. It is aided by a lower air temperature and by wind. A wind of 4 miles per hour is twice as effective in cooling as a wind of 1 mile per hour. (This is the basis for the wind-chill factor associated with winds in cool environments.)

Evaporation is the most effective method for cooling a body that is exercising in the air. The evaporation of sweat produces the cooling effect as perspiration goes from liquid to gas. This amounts to a cooling effect of over 580 kilocalories per liter of perspiration evaporated. This is enough heat to raise the temperature of 10 liters of water 58° C (10 ½ quarts of water 105° F). As the skin is cooled by the evaporation of sweat, it is able to take more of the heat from the blood and thereby cool the blood so that it can pick up more heat from the muscles.

The *hyperthermia* (high temperature) developed during exercise, particularly when the sweat cannot evaporate, is a major cause of fatigue. This is particularly true when the body has lost 2 percent of its water through perspiration. Since it is not uncommon to lose 1 to 5 liters of water while playing long hours in the hot sun, it is not difficult to enter the stage of *dehydration*. The combination of dehydration and high body temperature can cause a number of physiological problems, such as a reduction of blood volume, an increase in the breakdown of liver and muscle glycogen (a sugar used for muscle energy), and the inability of the body to effectively pass certain electrolytes across cell membranes.

A sudden change in the heat or humidity when you travel to a warmer or more humid climate to compete can cause problems. If you were to travel to India, Egypt, or the Caribbean to compete in a match, it would probably take ten days to two weeks to acclimatize yourself to the climate. Among the changes that will probably occur in the high heat are a reduced heart rate (due to less need for blood to heat the skin—resulting in less blood flow to the skin), an increase in the amount of blood plasma, increased sweating, perspiring earlier when exercising, increased salt losses, and the psychological adjustments made to the experience of greater heat and humidity.

Adequate fluid is essential to the functioning of an efficient body. When body fluids are reduced by sweating, less fluid is available in the blood and other tissues. This makes the body less efficient and, in some cases, can result in serious sickness or even death. To keep the body hydrated, you should take frequent breaks for fluid intake. However, even frequent breaks seldom give a tennis player enough fluid. Thirst does not signal the true need for fluids.

While it is recommended that people who exercise should replace 100 percent of the fluids lost, this is seldom done. The average person will replace only about 50 percent during the exercise period. Dehydration of 4 percent of the body's weight will reduce a person's endurance by 30 percent in temperate conditions, but as much as 50 percent when the weather is very warm.

The *ingredients of sweat* change as you exercise. At the beginning of exercise, your body excretes a number of salts. Sodium chloride (common table salt) as well as potassium, calcium, chromium, zinc, and magnesium salts can be lost. The initial sweat contains most of these salts, but as the exercise continues, the amount of salts in the sweat is reduced because some of the body's hormones come into play. Aldosterone, for example, conserves sodium for the body. Consequently, the longer you exercise, the more your sweat resembles pure water.

A normal diet replaces all of the necessary elements lost in sweat. Drinking a single glass of orange or tomato juice replaces all or most of the calcium, potassium, and magnesium lost. Further, most people have plenty of sodium in their daily diets.

Fluid-replacement drinks on the market are not necessarily recommended. Water, the most needed element, is slowed in its absorption if it contains other elements such as the salts and sugar in these drinks. Water alone is therefore generally the recommended fluid for fluid replacement—and it is certainly the least expensive. For those who, in addition to replacing water, want to replace sugars for energy, the best drinks are those containing glucose polymers (maltodextrins). So if you are using fluid-replacement drinks, check the label, then buy what you need—salts and/or sugars. Both caffeine (coffee, tea, and cola drinks) and alcohol dehydrate the body and should be avoided.

High humidity reduces the ability of your perspiration to be evaporated. Exercising in a rubber suit has similar effects to high humidity because the water cannot evaporate.

The best warm-weather clothing is no clothes. But unless you are playing in a nudist camp, you will have to wear something. Changing to dry clothes between matches is not advised because the evaporation effect is maximized when the clothing is wet.

Cold

Exercise in cold weather also requires adequate fluid intake. You must warm the air you breathe, your body is still producing heat, and you will tend to produce more urine. These factors require you to take in more fluid. If you don't, your body will feel colder because your blood will not have sufficient volume to warm your skin effectively with the heat it picks up from the exercising muscles.

Wind cools the body temperature faster than the registered temperature would warrant. We have all heard of the wind-chill factor present on colder days. The wind makes the body experience more cold than would be expected by the actual temperature. But even on warmer days, the wind will evaporate the perspiration and cool the body faster than might otherwise be expected. This may increase the need for fluids in order to continue the production of sweat.

Problems Caused by Heat

If you are concerned about overheating during your playing, it is recommended that you take your temperature with a rectal thermometer. Your temperature during and immediately after exercise should be below 104° F. Another type of thermometer would not give a true "core body" temperature because it would be affected by the cooling effects of sweating and other factors.

Heat Cramps

Heat cramps generally occur in the legs, arms, or abdomen. The victim will be able to think clearly and will have a normal rectal temperature. The treatment is to give fluids with salt and possibly other minerals, such as those found in most fluid-replacement drinks. Heat cramps are particularly common among exercisers who are not yet in good physical condition and who are participating in early workouts during warm days. There should be no problem in returning to activity the next day.

Heat Exhaustion

Heat exhaustion is generally caused by too little fluid or insufficient salts in the body.

Water-depletion heat exhaustion is caused by insufficient water intake or excessive sweating. The symptoms may include intense thirst, weakness, chills, fast breathing, impaired judgment, nausea, a lack of muscular coordination, and/or dizziness. If untreated, it can develop into heat stroke. The rectal temperature may be over 104° F (40° C). The skin will generally feel cool and somewhat moist. The immediate treatment is to give water or an electrolyte replacement drink. When the case is severe, it may require intravenous fluid replacement.

Salt-depletion heat exhaustion appears to be similar to heat cramps. This can occur when large volumes of sweat are replaced only with water. If a great deal of salt was lost in the perspiration, it can affect muscle functioning. It is most likely to occur during the first 5 to 10 days of exercising in the heat. The symptoms may include vomiting, nausea, inability to eat, diarrhea, a headache (particularly in the front of the head), weakness, a lower body temperature, and muscle cramps. Weight loss and thirst are not symptoms of this problem.

To prevent these heat-related problems, athletic trainers often require that athletes regain 80 percent of their fluid loss before leaving the locker room. So if an athlete weighed 150 pounds before practice and 146 pounds afterward, the trainer could require that the athlete take in enough fluids to bring the weight back to slightly over 149 pounds before leaving the facility.

Heat Stroke

Heat stroke can be caused by heavy exercise as well as by high air temperature. It is a very serious condition that can affect many of the organs. It can occur when the interior organs of the body are heated above 106° F (42° C). At this temperature, protein begins to break down. Enzymes are affected, as are the cell walls. When the cells cannot function effectively, the organ functioning is impaired.

In addition to a high body temperature, there may be a rapid pulse (100 to 120 beats per minutes) and low blood pressure. Other symptoms may include confusion, weakness, fatigue, or delirium, or the victim may lapse into a coma. The confusion that may be exhibited is often mistaken for a head injury in contact sports. The skin color is reddish, indicating poor circulation, and it will feel very hot and dry. There may or may not be sweating. The pupils of the eyes may be very small.

Treatment requires the immediate cooling of the body. Don't wait for the hospital to treat the victim. It may be too late. Use ice packs to the neck and groin. Full immersion in a tub of cold water is better. Anyone who has experienced a heat stroke should not return to activity for at least a week or two.

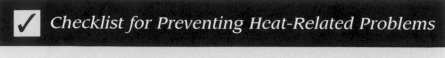

Checklist for Preventing Heat-Related Problems

1. Recognize the temperature and humidity and take the required measures to reduce injury.
2. Drink a great deal of water and possibly some fluid-replacement drinks during the practice, but don't take salt tablets. Drink more than you think you need. Drinks with a good deal of sugar may not be well tolerated by the body.
3. Wear cool clothing that allows the perspiration to escape—white clothes will reflect the sun better.
4. Exercise during the cooler part of the day—morning is better.

Summary

1. Playing long hours of tennis requires that you replace any nutrients that you lose.
2. Water is the most important nutrient to replace.
3. Sugars, particularly the quickly absorbed maltodextrins, aid in giving you quick energy by replacing the sugars that have been used for energy.
4. Fluid-replacement drinks may contain sugars and/or minerals (electrolytes).
5. You should be aware that heat-related injuries can occur on the tennis court and be able to recognize the symptoms.

Appendix

Tennis Resources

Simplified Rules of Tennis

To obtain a copy of the official rules of tennis, contact the USTA Bookstore:

USTA Bookstore
70 West Red Oak Lane
White Plains, NY 10604
(914) 696-7000, extension 6998

Joining a Tennis Association

To enhance your enjoyment of tennis, you might want to join a tennis association. You can join any group from a local recreation club or park league to the United States Tennis Association. Each group can keep you informed about tournaments and events in your area and each group can assist you in increasing your social contacts.

Local park groups and sectional associations connected with the United States Tennis Association (USTA) will provide you with the opportunity to increase your tennis skills, enter competitions, and meet other people with similar interests in tennis.

The United States Tennis Association

Applications for the United States Tennis Association can be obtained by writing:

USTA (United States Tennis Assn.)
70 W. Red Oak Lane
White Plains, NY 10604-3602

Memberships are available for adults, juniors, and families. There is also a life membership available.

Membership will include:

- A membership card, which is necessary for identifying yourself in many tournaments
- The opportunity to play in USTA-sanctioned tournaments and leagues
- A subscription to *World Tennis Magazine*
- A subscription to *Tennis USA*
- Discounts on tennis apparel and car rentals
- Discounts on USTA publications
- Consideration for ranking based on your tournament performances

In addition, local or sectional associations can:

- Sponsor tournaments
- Sponsor exhibitions
- Keep members informed on tournaments to watch
- Keep members informed on public appearances by leading professionals
- Sponsor clinics
- Organize special junior tournaments and clinics
- Organize instruction for underprivileged juniors
- Provide for "giveaways" of tennis equipment and supplies to the underprivileged
- Sponsor tennis tours in the United States and abroad for those interested in experiencing tennis around the world

Local and National Tennis Competition

Tennis competition is organized according to age and sex. There are age groups for boys and girls 12 years old and under, 14 and under, 16 and under, 18 and under, and 21 and under. A youth is eligible to compete in a certain age group as long as he or she has not yet reached the maximum age by the first of October in the year of competition.

Men's senior age groups are as follows: over 35, 50, 55, 60, 65, 70, 75, and 80. Women's groups are as follows: over 35, 40, 45, 50, 55, 60, 65, and 70. Adults are eligible for these senior groups if they will reach the minimum age for that group at any time during the year of competition.

Competition includes singles, doubles, and mixed doubles.

Glossary

Ace A serve that is hit so well that an opponent fails to touch it with his or her racket.

Ad Short for advantage; it is the first point scored after deuce. If the serving side scores, it is ad in; if the receiving side scores, it is ad out.

All An even score; a game score of 30 all, or a set score of 3 all, etc.

Alley The area outside the singles court that enlarges the width of the court for doubles. Each alley is 4 ½ feet wide.

American twist A serve in which the ball bounces high and in the opposite direction from which it was originally traveling.

Angle shot A ball hit to an extreme angle across the court.

Approach shot A ground stroke made while a player comes to the net.

Australian doubles Doubles in which the serve begins when the server and his or her partner are on the same half of the court.

Back court The area near the baseline.

Backhand The stroke used to return balls hit to the left side of a right-handed player.

Backhand court The left side of the court for a right-handed player.

Backspin Spin from top to bottom, applied by hitting down and through the ball; also called underspin. See also Chop; Slice.

Backswing The initial part of any swing; the act of bringing the racket back to prepare for the forward swing.

Ball boy A person who retrieves balls for tennis players during competition.

Baseline The end boundary line of a tennis court, located 39 feet from the net and paralleling the net.

Break point or break service To win a game in which an opponent serves.

Bye When a player is not required to play a particular round.

Cannonball A hard flat serve.

Center mark The short line that bisects the center of the baseline.

Center service line The line perpendicular to the net that divides the two service courts.

Center strap A strap in the center of the net, anchored to the ground to hold the net secure.

Chip A modified slice that requires a short swing; usually not hit hard; has underspin.

Choke To grip the racket higher on the handle than usual.

Chop A blocked spin shot that has more than the normal backspin; therefore, the racket moves down through the ball at a greater angle.

Closed face The angle of the hitting face of the racket when it is turned downward toward the court—the top edge of the racket head is forward of the bottom edge.

Consolation A tournament in which the loser continues to play in a losers' tournament.

Cross-court shot A shot in which the ball travels diagonally across the net, from one corner to the other.

Deep shot or depth A shot that bounces near the baseline, also near the service line on a serve.

Default Failure to complete a scheduled match in a tournament; such a player forfeits the match.

Deuce A tied score of at least 40–40 (the score is tied and each side has at least three points).

Deuce court Right court, so called because a deuce score is served there.

Dink A ball hit so it floats with extreme softness, usually very high.

Double elimination A tournament in which you must lose twice before you are eliminated.

Double-fault The failure of both service attempts to be good; results in loss of point.

Doubles A match with four players, two on each side.

Draw The means of establishing who plays whom in a tournament.

Drive A ground stroke hit with power.

Drop shot A softly hit shot that barely travels over the net.

Drop volley A drop shot that is hit from the volley position.

Earned point A point won by skillful playing rather than a player's mistake.

Elimination After being defeated in a tournament, one can no longer participate.

Error A point that ends in an obvious mistake.

Face The hitting surface of the racket.

Fast court A smooth-surfaced court that allows the ball to bounce quickly and low.

Fault An improper hit, generally thought of as a service error.

Fifteen The first point won by a player.

Flat shot A shot that travels in a straight line with little arc and little spin.

Floater A ball that moves slowly across the net in a high trajectory.

Foot fault A fault caused by the server stepping on or over the baseline before hitting the ball in service.

Force A ball hit with exceptional power; a play in which, because of the speed and placement of the shot, the opponent is pulled out of position.

Fore court The area between the net and service line.

Forehand court The right side of the court for a right-handed player.

Forty A player's score after winning three points.

Frame The part of the racket that holds the strings.

Game The part of a set that is completed when one player or side wins four points or two consecutive points after deuce.

Grip The method of holding the racket handle; the term given the leather covering on the handle.

Ground stroke Stroke made after the ball has bounced; either forehand or backhand.

Gut Racket strings made from animal intestines.

Half-volley Hitting the ball immediately after it bounces off the court.

Handle The part of the racket that is gripped in the hand.

Head The part of the racket used to hit the ball; includes the frame and strings.

Hold serve To serve and win that game.

Kill To smash the ball hard when hitting a winner.

Let A point played over because of interference; a serve that hits the top of the net but is otherwise good.

Linesman A person responsible for calling balls that land outside the court in competition.

Lob A ball hit high enough in the air to make the net-player reach up in order to hit the ball; usually hit high enough to go over the net-player's head.

Love Zero; no score.

Love game A game won without the loss of a point.

Love set A set won without the loss of a game.

Match Singles or doubles play that usually consists of two out of three sets; sometimes three out of five sets.

Match point The point that, if won, wins the match for the player.

Midcourt The area in the center of the playing court, midway between the net and the baseline.

Mix up To vary the types of shots selected.

Net game To play the net; also called net play.

Net-player The partner in doubles who plays at the net.

No man's land Midcourt, where many balls bounce at the player's feet.

Open face The hitting face of the racket when it is turned up away from the court surface—with the bottom edge of the racket head ahead of the top edge.

Opening A mistake that allows an opponent a good chance to score a point.

Out A ball landing outside the playing area.

Overhead smash See Smash.

Overspin See Topspin.

Pace Speed; usually refers to the speed of a ball.

Passing shot A ground stroke hit; made in an attempt to hit out of the reach of a net-player.

Percentage tennis Cutting down on unnecessary errors.

Place To hit the ball to an intended area.

Placement A shot hit so that an opponent cannot reach it.

Poach When the net-player in doubles moves over to his or her partner's side of the court to make a volley.

Point The part of a game started by a serve and ended when a player or side wins or misses a shot.

Press A wooden or metal frame that holds a tennis racket firmly enough to prevent warping.

Rally Hitting the ball back and forth over the net a number of times; can occur in practice or matches.

Retrieve To return a very difficult shot.

Round robin A tournament in which every player plays every other player.

Rush To move to the net after hitting a shot.

Seed To arrange a tournament so that the top players don't play against each other until the final rounds.

Serve (service) The shot that starts a point.

Service line The line that is parallel to and 21 feet from the net.

Set The part of the match that is completed when one player or side wins at least six games and is ahead by at least two games, or when one player has won the tiebreaker.

Set point The point that, if won, will win the set.

Side spin A shot that, when hit, spins to the side and bounces to the side.

Singles A match between two players.

Slice A shot hit with backspin; your racket hits the ball when traveling down through the ball. This shot has less spin and more power than the chip or chop.

Slow court A court, such as a soft court made of dirt or clay, that makes the ball bounce slower and higher.

Smash A hard shot hit at the net, usually an overhead shot.

Spin Hitting the ball at an angle, causing the ball to rotate in an unusual manner; see Topspin; Sidespin; Slice; Backspin.

Straight sets To win a match without the loss of a set.

Sweet spot The area in the center of strings of the racket where the truest shot can be made.

Tape The white band that runs across the top of the net.

Tennis elbow A condition in the elbow caused by undue pressure or strain; common to tennis players and very painful.

Thirty The second point won by the player in a game.

Throat The part of the racket between the handle and the head.

Tiebreaker An official nine-point, twelve-point, or thirteen-point sudden-death scoring system when the score is tied at six games all.

Topspin Spin of the ball from top to bottom, caused by hitting up and through the ball; it makes the ball bounce high and fast.

Trajectory The angle of the ball in relation to its contact with the racket, and the flight of the ball over the top of the net, such as a high or low trajectory.

Umpire The person who officiates at matches.

Undercut See Backspin; Chip; Chop; Slice.

Underspin See Backspin; Chip; Chop; Slice.

Unseeded Those players who are not favored to win a tournament; they are not given any special placing in the draw.

VASSS Van Alen Simplified Scoring System A 31-point scoring system.

Volley To hit the ball before it bounces.

Wood shot A ball hit on the frame of the racket.

Index